PRAISE FOR

HOODOO HERBAL

"Filled with down-home charm, essential Bible verses, recipes, valuable herb, plant, and root correspondences, and a whole lot of real talk, *Hoodoo Herbal* should be explored by every aspiring conjure worker. The passing along of practical information is essential to the history and preservation of any craft, and Starr Casas shines brightly here in the sharing of her knowledge and lived conjure experiences."

—Cairelle Crow, owner of Sacred Roots and editor of
Brigid's Light

"Mama Starr did it again! Her *Hoodoo Herbal* contains herbal techniques that she has previously only ever shared in person or through her private classes. Much of the information found here will not be found anywhere else. As with all of her other works, Mama Starr makes sure that her readers know where this work comes from and the importance of keeping the Bible in the work. The works presented are authentic and powerful. As she says early on in the book, in Conjure work, the work is the work. Anyone interested in Conjure/Rootwork and looking for an herbal resource, this book is it. Highly recommended for anyone interested in herbal folklore."

—Charity Bedell, author of *Container Magic* and coauthor
of *The Good Witch's Guide: A Modern-Day Wiccapedia of
Magickal Ingredients and Spells* (Volume 2)

"My bookshelves swell with books by Starr Casas and for good reasons. They give the reader authentic lore, powerful workings, and practical teachings fueled by an uncompromising commitment to the work's elders, ancestors, and cultures. They reflect a clarity that only comes through a genuine living folk tradition. With *Hoodoo Herbal*, Starr Casas has produced an outstanding compendium of lore, recipes, prayers, Bible passages, spells, allied spirits, and other practices, all steeped in the depth, potency, practicality, and authenticity of living folk magic—the hallmark of all her works. She shares the power of what my Momma called "Eden's Eldest Children": herbs, other plants, their uses and preparations in Conjure and Rootwork. But Starr's book goes beyond the usual offerings of plant magic books to include potent time-honored techniques that awaken and increase the spirit and the power. This is what makes the work really work!"

—Orion Foxwood, author of
Mountain Conjure and Southern Root Work

"Starr Casas does it again! In *Hoodoo Herbal*, she provides a complete foundation and working knowledge of some of the most important components of Hoodoo and Conjure: herbs. Plants are at the foundation of most magical practices, especially Hoodoo. This book empowers the reader to have the knowledge of using these essential items in a way that creates massive change. A must-read."

—Hector Salva, author of
The 21 Divisions and *Espiritismo*

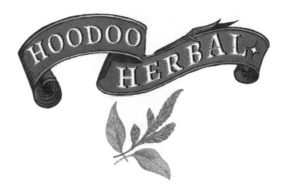

STARR CASAS

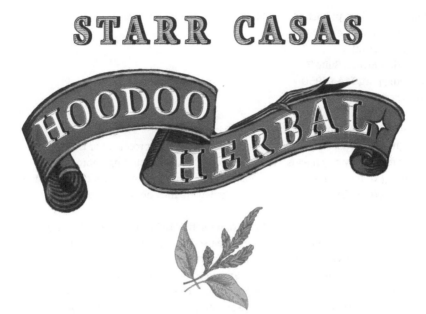

HOODOO HERBAL

Folk Recipes for Conjure & Spellwork
with Herbs, Houseplants,
Roots & Oils

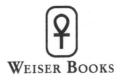

WEISER BOOKS

This edition first published in 2022 by Weiser Books, an imprint of
Red Wheel/Weiser, LLC
With offices at:
65 Parker Street, Suite 7
Newburyport, MA 01950
www.redwheelweiser.com

This book contains advice and information relating to herbs and is not meant
to diagnose, treat, or prescribe. It should be used to supplement, not replace, the
advice of your physician or other trained healthcare practitioner. If you know or
suspect you have a medical condition, are experiencing physical symptoms, or
if you feel unwell, seek your physician's advice before embarking on any medical program or treatment. Some of the substances discussed in this book can
be lethal if mishandled or ingested in sufficient quantities. Extreme caution is
advised in their handling and use. Readers are also cautioned to follow all instructions carefully and accurately for safety and the best effect. Readers using the
information in this book do so entirely at their own risk, and the author and pub-
lisher accept no liability if adverse effects are caused.

ISBN: 978-1-57863-785-0
Library of Congress Cataloging-in-Publication Data available upon request.

Cover design by Kathryn Sky-Peck
Interior by Maureen Forys, Happenstance Type-O-Rama
Typeset in Macklin Slab, Sovereign Display

Printed in the United States of America
IBI
10 9 8 7 6 5 4 3 2 1

*This book is dedicated
to all my elders.*

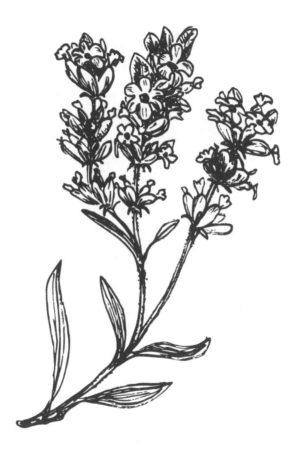

CONTENTS

CONTENTS

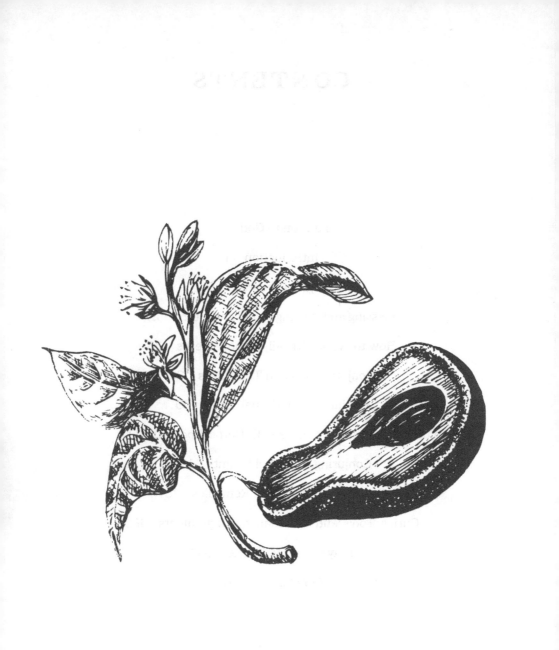

PETITION TO GOD

I Petition Thee, God on high and the almighty spirits that walk with you Lord. I come to you in prayer and petition that you will remove all crossed conditions that may be affecting my life. Remove them with your mighty hand. I ask this in the name of God the FATHER, God the SON, and the God the HOLY SPIRIT, Amen.

I Petition THE HOLY TRINITY. Please remove all blocks and cross conditions that may be affecting me and mine. I ask this in the name of God the FATHER, God the SON, and the God the HOLY SPIRIT, Amen.

I petition Thee, SAINT MICHAEL, GOD'S RIGHT-HAND MAN, sever all ties to ALL my enemies known, unknown, hidden, ALIVE & DEAD that work against me day and night, dark and light. Destroy all crossed conditions that bind my spirit. With your mighty Sword cut all ties to ALL my enemies! Amen.

I Pray that the HOLY TRINITY will protect me and shield me against all my enemies; I pray for the gift of Discernment so I may know them by the darkness of their spirit. I pray the Trinity will gift me with the Spirit of Truth and Wisdom so that I may always see what is hidden and done in the dark so it may be brought to light. I pray this in the name of God the Father, God the Son, God the Holy Spirit, and in the name of the Ancestors. Amen.

I call on my Ancestors, Known and Unknown, BLOOD OF MY BLOOD, and all the spirits that walk with me. I ask that you protect and defend me against all those who would harm me or mine. I pray that every hit be returned tenfold in the name of God the Father, God the Son, and God the Holy Spirit, the Ancestors and all the spirits that walk with me. Amen.

I cover this prayer and my petition with the blood of Jesus! I cover my enemies and any works they have laid against me with the blood of Jesus; may it burn and be destroyed! I call on the Holy Trinity to guard me and keep me and mine safe! AMEN.

INTRODUCTION

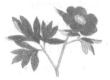

Like most of my books, this book has been in the making for about seven years. As everyone who reads my writings knows, I tend to do things my own way and follow my own spirits. When I picked this book back up, I already had quite a few pages written. That is one of my bad habits as a writer: I'll start a book, and then for whatever reason I'll put it down, then come back to it later and pick it back up.

I wanted this book to be special and to touch on all parts of working with roots and herbs, whether you're cooking dinner or putting together conjure work or a medicinal brew. I feel that the culture of Conjure is changing as more outsiders come in and try to make it fit their lifestyles. I wanted to draw folks back into the traditions that this work comes from.

Herbs play a large part in conjure works. The properties herbs and roots hold are the foundation of conjure oils, powders, washes, candles and conjure bags along with candles and prayers. The reason many conjure workers are called rootworkers or root doctors is because roots and herbs are such a big part of their work.

Conjure oils are worked with to feed and empower the work and the ingredients that make up the work. There are many oils that are worked with as base oils such as olive oil and mineral oil. These are also called anointing oils or dressing oils—it depends on if you are talking to an outsider or someone from the culture.

You will find all types of conjure information here relating to herbs and oils, plus workings with houseplants and herbal remedies and all types of Southern dishes that I grew up on. The thing that needs to be remembered is the conjure worker back in the time of slavery knew how to curse and cure, how to heal with food and how to cross. I've never really shared this much before, but I see folks online hinting at it so I decided just to put it out there.

This book is going to be organized a little differently than my other books. We are going to look at the various types of plants and how they work in Conjure, and that is our focus. But I will bring in more information and works as we go along. I'll talk about some conjure essentials to get you started and add in works as they come up.

There is a lot of useful and helpful information in this book. I read somewhere that someone said that today's conjure books are full of nothing but recipes with the spirit of the work missing. I have to totally disagree. Conjure work is putting ingredients together that hold power and can get the job done. To be very clear conjure work *is* the work. Yes, we all have a spiritual side to us, but this work is all about the roots, herbs, curios, and ingredients that go into the packets, the conjure bags, the medicine bottles, and the power of the prayers and petitions—it really doesn't have much to do with the worker's spiritual side. The most spiritual side of this work is the Christian aspects of working with the Bible within traditional Conjure—the

Trinity, the books of the Bible, the spirituals, and the prayers and petition that are a central part of the works.

I know some folks tend to take a work and try to make it fit them. The thing with Conjure is that it comes from a whole culture that grew up in the South over years and years and extreme circumstances that we can't even imagine today, so when folks try to change a work, they are trying to either add to or remove something from the culture. I say if it ain't broke, don't try to fix it. Either do the work the way it's supposed to be done or find something that suits your spirit better. In this book, I will give you tools to do things the way my family has always done them.

I hope you enjoy this book as much as I have enjoyed writing it.

From the Heart

Conjure is a living culture; it has not died out nor does it need to be revamped. It's engrained in Southern folks from the time they are old enough to understand; although it isn't called by any name, it is what we are taught as young children. It may be a little different depending on what area you come from, but the foundation will always be similar. Southern children are taught from an early age how to act in public: what to say, what not to say. We are taught to be polite even if you can't stand someone. (This is where terms like "bless their heart" comes from: that phrase is a blessing and insult all wrapped up in one and is said with a sweet voice.) In order to really understand the work, you need to understand the folks who brought the work here.

There's a big difference between looking in through a window and working with someone from that culture and being part of the Southern culture. It's a way of life that's "lived daily" by Southern folk. This culture is a lot more than oils, powders, baths, or "spells"—as an outsider would call the work. It is a way of thinking; a way of moving through life. I guess you could say it is a mindset. I have spoken with many folks over the years that come from the South even though they may live somewhere else now; nine times out of ten we have some common thread even though we were raised by different families and in different areas.

I can't speak for city folks in the South because my people come from the rural areas. I can only speak of what I know or have been taught. Southern folks don't just start spouting out information; they want to know who they are speaking to. Most will ask about your people upon meeting you. This is one reason I feel the Hyatt works you can find in his books and online that so many people think are the be-all and end-all of Conjure are mostly old wives' tales. If you went running around the rural South spouting off about "spells," you might be run off with the end of a shotgun!

Most of this started with the Harry Middleton Hyatt books on Hoodoo and Conjure, where folks shared information with Hyatt, who was collecting folklore. I have never tried to keep my strong opinion of Hyatt a secret. I have a few issues with the Hyatt material, but I think my main issue, the more I study his book 1, is the disrespect I'm seeing for the workers trying to share their information with him. He doesn't let them finish what they are telling until he moves them on to something else. To me, most of the information is half-baked cakes. Some of it in those books is just enough to get you in trouble—especially the stuff dealing with the dead and graveyards.

Reading about something and living it are two different things. Understanding a culture and growing up in it every day of your life are also two different things. Southern folks have a whole different way of looking at life than folks from other places. This work has been passed down from one family member to the next or from an elder; it was not out in the public. The work was a very well-kept secret; it was all done in a day of family life. Whatever came along, there was a way to help from illness to nightmares, hag riding, and such.

This work was never meant to be advertised and spread around like chicken feed. This work was shared hands-on; it was passed down from an elder. Before I got online you only came to me if one of my clients sent you. Folks didn't have big ole signs out everywhere; you might find one or two small ones advertising treatments and such. It was a community base where folks knew where to go when they needed something. Conjure was and is for the community the worker lives in.

I never advertised, I still don't not really. I have found the adjustment hard at times but I have stuck with it and I have become well known in my circle outside of my community. Through word of mouth folks know who I am. There's more to this work than just the works; there is a whole culture blended into it. It is part of the works from the way we bathe to the way we sweep.

For example, I was taught to sweep the yard at a very young age. My grandmamma didn't tell me why; she showed me how. Back then everyone swept their yards. When I was young, folks had a routine.

It wasn't odd because everyone did the same thing at some point during the week and most did the work at the same time.

Brooms and sweeping are a big thing in conjure work. As most know, it is done to remove unwanted things. Sweeping is a way of cleansing, and cleansing work is a large part of Conjure. I was taught growing up how it fits in what the world today calls Hoodoo, Conjure, and Rootwork. My grandma made her own brooms to sweep the yards with. And I say "yards" because the front yard and backyard were considered to be separate.

Nowadays folks don't have to sweep their yards, but they do rake them and raking falls right in line with sweeping; it is all cleaning. My point is that just the way children in the South are taught to sweep is the same concept in Conjure for doing cleansing work. If you are doing a house cleansing, you would start at the back of the house and work forward to the front; if you are doing a cleansing on the body, you would start at the crown of the head and go downward and outward just like you would if you were sweeping. This is where the foundation is built.

Like I have said over and over, it is a culture, a way of life that you grow up with. Still, I think everyone has a right to practice Conjure if they are called to do the work and remember to honor the elders this work comes from.

My best advice is to find an elder and learn all you can. It won't take you long to see the real deal from the pieced-together bits. Take your time; really try to understand the mindset of the rural folks of the South where this work really comes from. Read all you can read and use discernment to see what is real and what isn't. Some of these works are hidden in plain sight. It's like in the old spirituals: there is work in those spirituals but you have to be able to see it.

This book is a collection of works to help folks learn or just to share my culture with other folks before it is lost. It's my hope it is a useful book and might help someone.

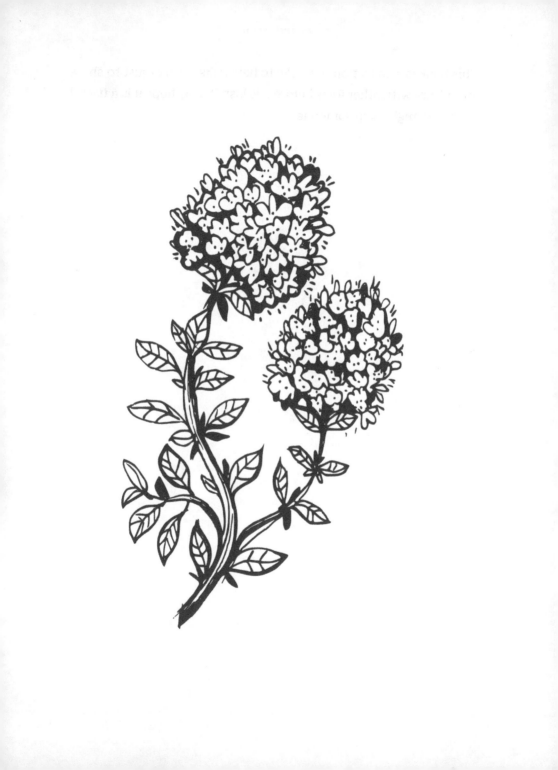

CONJURE ESSENTIALS

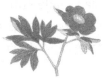

I'm not going to spend a lot of time on the essentials of Conjure. I've done that in my other books. But I will give you some information here on what you need to know to understand Conjure and the works that come up in this book.

The Bible

The Holy Bible—and the Old Testament especially—is the foundation of conjure work. I was not taught to work with the New Testament, so all my teachings I share with my students to work with are from the Old Testament.

It seems to me that when Conjure was first introduced on the internet, folks failed to introduce the Bible that goes along with the work. I know a lot of folks would prefer that the Bible be left completely out, but once you do that, you are no longer doing Conjure. It can be debated and has been debated to death about whether the Bible is needed in conjure work, but the fact remains that the Old Testament of the Bible is worked to help draw power into works.

There are those who wish Conjure wasn't Christian, but the Trinity and the Bible are a large part of conjure work. Why would you take the power away from the work you're doing? That doesn't make any kind of sense. If you are going to do conjure work, then work with the Bible. The power of the work is hidden within the pages. Forget about the man-made churches and all the hogwash so-called Christians have spewed out that have turned you away. Learn the work the right way, and don't throw the baby out with the bathwater!

On the other side of things, I have been attacked for teaching non-Christians Conjure. Some folks have gone so far as to say that if you're not a Christian, then you have no place in Conjure. I highly disagree with that. No one has the right to tell another person what they can and cannot do within their own religious beliefs. The only thing I care about is this work living on and being done the way the elders have taught it.

The Old Testament is full of works that can be used to help yourself or a client. And not only are the scriptures a part of the work, but the Catholic saints and prophets are also petitioned in the work. I work with my ancestors, some saints, and the prophets. And on the subject of plants, the herbs and oils that were worked with in the Bible can add great power to work.

Did you know that hyssop—a member of the mint family—is considered a holy herb. Hyssop is one of the most potent herbs in the Old Testament. It is alleged to add great power to when worked with for cleansing, protection, and purification.

In Bible times many doctors and folks collecting dead bodies were covered in it. And when the black plague was running rampant in Europe, hyssop was used to dress the inside of masks to keep folks from inhaling the smell and the disease. Exodus 12:22 tells us, "And ye shall take a bunch of hyssop, and dip it in the blood that is in the bason, and strike the lintel and the two side posts with the blood that is in the bason; and none of you shall go out at the door of his house until morning." This was done for protection, and some elders say that this verse will stop excessive bleeding.

Psalm 51 V 7 says, "Cleanse me with hyssop, and I will be clean; wash me, and I will be whiter than snow." This verse tells us that hyssop will help in all cleansing work. It will help with any condition such as cleansing, uncrossing, blockbuster works, or even jinx removing.

If you look at Genesis 30 V 14–16, you see that mandrake was used for love and money in the Old Testament or as a tool to barter with.

14 In the days of wheat harvest Reuben went and found mandrakes in the field and brought them to his mother Leah. Then Rachel said to Leah, "Please give me some of your son's mandrakes."

15 But she said to her, "Is it a small matter that you have taken away my husband? Would you take away my son's mandrakes also?" Rachel said, "Then he may lie with you tonight in exchange for your son's mandrakes."

16 When Jacob came from the field in the evening, Leah went out to meet him and said, "You must come in to me, for I have hired you with my son's mandrakes." So he lay with her that night.

Mandrake root is worked with for love, power, and money-drawing conjures.

Some of the other herbs used for baths and holy oils were balm of Gilead, camphor, saffron, and cinnamon.

Here is a small list of biblical herbs and the scriptures they can be found in. This is by no means all of them. There are a lot of interesting works that can be found in the Bible, like I was taught. Always keep in mind the Bible is of God; churches are of man!

Anise (Matthew 23 V 23)

Balm of Gilead (Jeremiah 46 V 11)

Coriander (Exodus 16 V 31; Numbers 11 V 7)

Cinnamon (Exodus 30 V 23; Revelation 18 V 13)

Cumin (Isaiah 28 V 25; Matthew 23 V 23)

Dill (Matthew 23 V 23)

Garlic (Numbers 11 V 5)

Mint (Matthew 23 V 23; Luke 11 V 42)

Mustard (Matthew)

Rue (Luke 11 V 42)

In the time of the Bible folks always had pots and containers filled with herbs, tinctures, and holy oils. It was a way of life for them. Most old-school workers continue to keep pots and containers of things needed for the work.

The Altar

The altar is *the* foundation of your spiritual work. It is the crossroads where you meet Spirit. It is a place where you can speak to your God and ancestors. It's a place of power.

Prayer

When you pray your petitions, you are opening the way for Spirit to come forth and answer those prayers and petitions. It is important to always pray from the heart. Later in this book, I will share more about prayers from the Old Testament so you can have a better idea of what these look like.

For now, one of my favorite prayers from the Bible is Psalm 23.

> *Psalm 23 V 1-6*
>
> *1 The Lord is my shepherd; I shall not want.*
>
> *2 He maketh me to lie down in green pastures: he leadeth me beside the still waters.*
>
> *3 He restoreth my soul: he leadeth me in the paths of righteousness for his name's sake.*
>
> *4 Yea, though I walk through the valley of the shadow of death, I will fear no evil: for thou art with me; thy rod and thy staff they comfort me.*
>
> *5 Thou preparest a table before me in the presence of mine enemies: thou anointest my head with oil; my cup runneth over.*
>
> *6 Surely goodness and mercy shall follow me all the days of my life: and I will dwell in the house of the Lord for ever.*

Petitions

A petition is basically a way of putting your words into a prayer. These petitions are prayed by calling on the Trinity, your ancestors, and any other spirit you might be calling upon for help. One thing that you have to remember is that you have to be very clear when you are petitioning Spirit. Words hold power. And Spirit takes your words directly to heart. That's what makes praying your petition to Spirit so powerful while doing your work.

The Ancestors

You should always call on the Trinity first, and then your ancestors, then the spirit you are going to be working with other than the Trinity or your ancestors. Our ancestors should be a very important part of our lives. Everyone should have a small space set up for their ancestors where they can honor them at least once a week. After all, if it weren't for them, none of us would be here.

It doesn't matter what day in the week; you can choose whichever day works best for you. Offer your ancestors a cool glass of water, a small candle, and say some prayers in their honor.

Another way to honor them is by going to the graveyard and cleaning their graves. This is part of the Southern culture. Dressing and cleansing headstones honor our dead. Their graves should never be allowed to become overgrown and disheveled—this is very disrespectful.

Candles

While candles are more of a tool than an essential, I'll tell you about them now because they are central in so many of the works that follow. Candles have been burned since the days of the Old Testament either in the form of a pillar or an oil lamp. The flames draw power and bring forth spirits that can be very helpful in the work.

The color of the candle can be important. Use this list to help you determine what color you need for a work.

Red heats up any conjure work.

Orange adds power to workings.

Green is used with Saint Martha Conjure as well as money and luck workings.

Blue is used for peaceful home and money Conjure, as well as court case works.

Purple is a very powerful color in Conjure used for wisdom, controlling, and power strengthening.

Black is used for cleansings, reversals, and jinx removing. It also absorbs evil and keeps the devil running.

White is used for cleansing, healing, and peace workings. It is also used for drawing truth and spiritual power into Conjure.

Gray represents the area between the spirit world and the physical realm. As a mixture of black and white, it is a powerful conjure color for working with Spirit as well as uncrossing works.

Spiritual Discernment

The Hierarchy in Traditional Old Style Conjure should be the Holy Trinity first, your Ancestors and then any other Spirit you choose with.

—*HOODOO MONEY CONJURE* by Mama Starr Casas

Spiritual discernment is being able to see everything that is going on within the spiritual realm whether it is doing a reading or working with a client. You have to be able to read Spirit—which is actually what spiritual discernment is.

Anytime you do any type of prayer or power work, you are drawing all kinds of spirits and things that you can't see, whether they are good or bad, and you are opening yourself up to them. Just like folks you deal with in everyday life, the spirits you come in contact with have their own motives for being around you. It's very important that you be able to discern what has drawn a spirit to you and what exactly they want from you. Another good rule I was taught as a young worker was to never go searching a spirit out. If you are meant to work with them, they will lead you to them.

You should never just jump in with both feet and work with a spirit blindly. That is very, very dangerous. I know folks won't necessarily listen to this advice, but like my mama always told us, "a hard head makes a soft behind!" Discernment of Spirit is a very important key to being a successful conjure worker. It not only helps you to see the spirits that are around you, but being able to discern what's happening in the spiritual world will save you from many trials and tribulations. In order to find a crossed condition, you have to be able to discern what Spirit is trying to tell you.

The first step in developing spiritual discernment is to learn to *listen* to what Spirit is saying. Pay attention in the emotions you feel, the voice that you hear, or the heaviness or lightness of Spirit. Another thing that is really important is to know which spirit is speaking to you: your own or the spirits that walk with you. Know the difference between your own voice and the voice of Spirit because without that you're just spinning your wheels.

The Bible tells us that we should always test any spirits that we are in communication with to make sure they are who they claim to be. The best way to do this is to first ask questions that you already know the answers to. This way you can tell if they are being truthful or not. Do not be gullible enough to think that you control the spirits.

Here is a listing of the different types of spirits that you could possibly run into in your work, but this is by no means all of them.

Intranquil Spirits

The intranquil spirit is a type that seems to be popular nowadays. The thing that I don't think most folks understand is that this spirit will take total control and suck the life out of you. I'm not trying to scare you or put fear in you. I'm just telling it like it is. There are many of these intranquil spirits. It is not just one spirit that you are dealing with.

Caution should always be used when dealing with any type of spirit, but especially this spirit, which is a demon—or I should say those spirits which are demons. I can't caution you enough to leave these types of spirits alone.

Vengeful Spirits

Vengeful spirits are no saints. They are full of rage and hate. These spirits died from extreme causes, or they could just have been evil when they were walking the earth. Once again, this is not the type of spirit that you want to call on or petition to help you. This is the type of spirit that will turn on you in a heartbeat and they are not to be trusted. Use your common sense and leave this type of spirit alone.

There is no reason to work with this spirit because you can call on your ancestors instead to avenge or set straight a wrong that has been done to you.

Graveyard Spirits

Folks just love going to the graveyard and playing around. Everybody loves working with the spirits of the graveyard. The problem with that is if you are not trained or you just read something somewhere and decided to try it out, then you are opening yourself up to a whole lot of trouble. These spirits can work for you or against you. Unless they are your blood kin, you really don't know what you are getting, and even with your blood kin you are taking a chance. I've said this over and over again: no one should be working with a graveyard spirit that they do not know because you don't have a clue of what type of person that spirit was in life. You are taking a chance of that spirit turning on you.

Demons & Djinn

I really don't know anything about the djinn except for what Rosemary Ellen Guiley shared on the *Old Style Conjure* radio show with me. I understand that the djinn and demons come from the same family. I also understand that the djinn are really tricky and should be left alone. Like some folks they are two-faced and only show you the side they want you to see until the game is up. Only then will they show their true selves!

You should always do what is best for you. You should never follow behind anyone blindly. If you want to work in the graveyard, then please find an elder who is willing to teach you hands-on graveyard work. And work with your ancestors for a few years to get to know them. There is no rush. It has taken me over half my life to get where I am today, and I am still learning new things. It is much safer to work with your ancestors, the saints, and the prophets than it is to mess with unknown spirits. This way you are covered by the power of God and your ancestors rather than messing with something that you know nothing about. For prayers and petitions to these safe spirits, see that chapter at the back of this book.

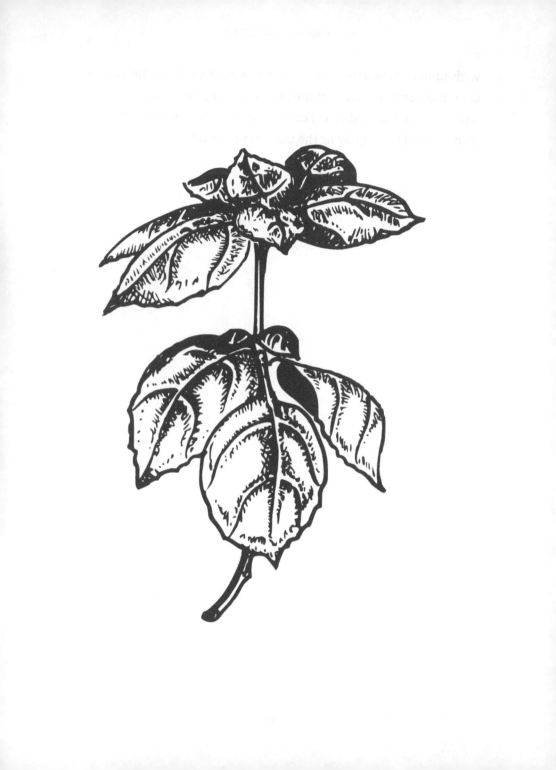

BLESSING AND WAKING ROOTS AND HERBS

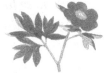

Anything that is a living plant has life. Conjure workers have been working with roots and herbs for hundreds of years. There is an herbal remedy for every single ailment, whether the problem needs a medicinal or a spiritual cure. Countryfolk tend to depend more on roots and herbs for remedies than city folk do. When I was a child, my mama treated us with old sayings, prayer, and remedies. We didn't go to the doctor: she was our doctor. Folks like my mama were well-respected for their knowledge of healing. Nowadays most folks buy their roots and herbs from stores; very few harvest their own.

You can't just throw some ingredients together for them to do what you want. To work with plants, you need to bless and wake them.

Blessing Roots and Herbs

Place your ingredients in a triangle setup of white candles, and then say your blessing prayer over them at least three times.

Herbal Blessing

> *I call on God the Father, God the Son, and God the Holy Spirit; I call on my ancestors!*
>
> *I petition you to wake up these herbs, roots, and curios so they will bring forth their full power and add it to the work.*
>
> *I call on the Trinity and my Ancestors, may you add your power to these ingredients with your power!*
>
> *I ask this in the name of God the Father, God the Son, and God the Holy Spirit. Amen.*

Waking Up the Roots

One of the most important things you need to do when you have a conjure job to do is gather up the roots and herbs you will be working with and work them first. You can't just throw a bunch of roots and herbs into a work and expect them to do their job. Not much will happen in that work.

You need to *feed* your ingredients before they are added to your work. By feeding them you are waking up the spirit of the root or herb. You will need a white hankie, five tealights, and a little whiskey to do this. Lay out the hankie and put the ingredients in the center.

Place four of the tealights in a cross setup around them, and then place the last tealight on top of the mixture. Light the tealights, and say your prayers and petitions over the mixture. Go back often to pray over the work as the lights burn.

Once the lights go out, gather up the hankie and hold it close to your mouth, praying your petition and prayers into the hankie. Then spread the hankie out again, repeat the prayers and petition, and sprinkle the ingredients with whiskey. I like to place the ingredients in another setup and say prayers and petitions until the lights go out. Then I will add the ingredients into the rest of the work.

You should repeat this process with all the ingredients that will be going into the work. The more they are empowered with prayer, the stronger the work will be. I know it seems like a lot to do, but in the long run it will be worth it.

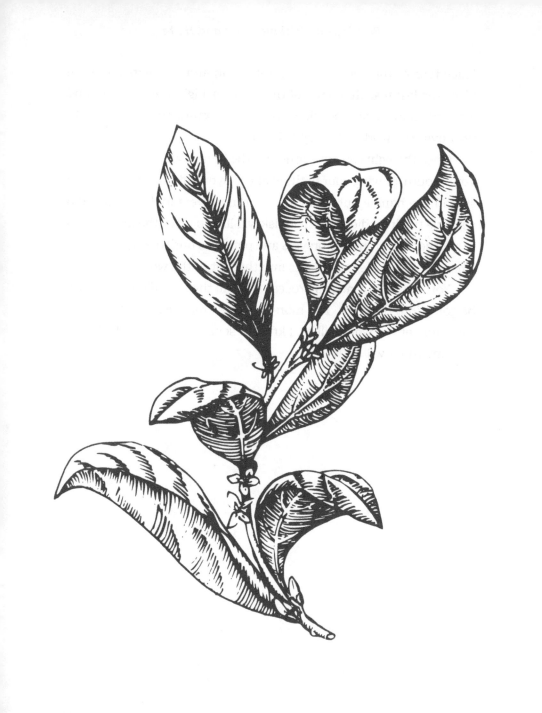

HOW TO WORK WITH ALL-PURPOSE HERBS

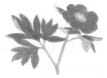

There are many herbs and roots that have a dual purpose. As a worker it is your job to know how to work with them. If you look in the herbal section of this book, you will see that the herbs and roots are listed as cold, hot, or dual. The information is right at your fingertips with easy access to what you may be looking for. I'm gonna list a few here as examples, so you get a feel for this. The herbs listed below will be able to draw as well as repel.

Basil (dual)

Basil is worked for all money matters. It is also said to strengthen the love and happiness within the home. Basil works for sending evil away. It is a good herb to add to all run devil run works. For protection, get a bundle of fresh basil and hang it inside your front door. As it dries, you can work with it as a broom and brush yourself off daily.

Broomstraw (dual)

Broomstraw can be worked with for protection and cleansing. The old folks say that it will sweep away evil and witches. It can also be worked for crossing and jinxing.

Irish Moss (dual)

Irish moss is worked with to draw prosperity and also for protection. Irish moss can also be worked with all types of crossing work; that is one of the reasons that it is a dual herb.

Peony Root (dual)

Peony root can break old jinxes and draw forth good fortune. It is said to help the wearer against misfortune, but it can also be worked to bring misfortune on a target.

These are just a few examples. You can see how these herbs can work both sides of an issue: this is where your prayers and petitions play even a larger part in your work. You will need to be very clear in your petition. There are many more all-purpose herbs, and you'll see a few of them in the main herb list. Just remember all work should be justified lest you be hit with your own work.

Heat It Up or Cool It Down

There are times when you need to either cool down a work or heat it up. There are many herbs and roots that can be found to help you do just that. In the herbal section of the book, you will find that each root or herb listed is identified as cool, hot, or dual. Cool and hot are self-explanatory, and dual means the root or herb goes both ways like we just looked at.

If you need to heat a work up, I have found it easiest to get an herb that is hot and goes along with whatever the work is. Here is a short list to get you started.

Love Works

Ginseng Root (hot)

Ginseng root is worked with in all types of money and gambling jobs. It is a very hot root and is worked with in all types of work to add heat. It is also said to enhance male vigor.

Juniper Berries (hot)

These are worked with to attract love. It is said when a woman carries them in a packet, they will draw a lover to her.

Money Works

Cloves (hot)

Cloves are worked with in some shut your mouth work, but they are well-known for the power that they bring to all conjure works for prosperity and better business.

Fenugreek Seed (hot)

Mama Starr loves this stuff! It is worked for drawing money and luck into your home. Add fenugreek seeds to a small white bowl with a pinch of sugar and some shredded money. Place this high in the kitchen on top of the icebox. This is a trick of Mama Starr's to keep prosperity coming into her home.

Protection Works

Devil Pod (hot)

This pod is worked with for a strong protection against evil and any dark spirits sent to harm you by an enemy. Get a small devil pod and feed it whiskey, then place it in a candle setup. Once the candles burn out, place the pod in a red flannel bag and carry it at your waist, or if you're a woman, you can carry it in your bosom.

Devil's Shoestring (hot)

Devil's shoestring comes in handy within all enemy work. Three devil's shoestrings tied together with your photo in the center of them is strong protection and will send the devil running. Devil's shoestrings are also used in all works to nail the devil down.

If you need to cool a target or a situation down, you can add one of the roots or herbs to the work.

Healing Works

Coltsfoot (cool)

Coltsfoot can be added to a spiritual wash to remove illness from a sickroom. It is also said that it can be mixed with other herbs to bring forth psychic visions.

Eyebright (cool)

Eyebright is a healing herb first and foremost. If you are having issues with your eyes, a cool bath of eyebright will help soothe them.

Eyebright is also worked with in Conjure to see what is hidden and also to help the worker see clearly.

Feverfew (cool)

Feverfew is worked with as a wash to be added to a tub of cool water to relieve a fever. It is also added to protection for folks who tend to always end up being harmed or hurt in accidents.

Peaceful Home Works

Borage Flowers (cool)

These flowers are effective in all types of peaceful home workings. They are believed to calm hotheads and to bring peace to the target.

Lavender (cool)

Lavender is worked with in peaceful home works. Lavender soothes and cools down the spirit. It works wonders for folks who are hot-headed or bullheaded.

Lovage (dual)

Lovage is worked with in all love works. It is wonderful when you are working on yourself; it promotes self-love and a high self-esteem. In washes or sprinkled around the home, it brings love and peace to the home.

Sweetening Works

Honeysuckle (cool)

Honeysuckle is worked with in all types of sweetening work. The vine of the honeysuckle can be wrapped around a photo of you and your lover to draw you closer together and to sweeten the love you have for each other.

Jasmine Flowers (cool)

Jasmine is worked with in all types of love work; it is also said that jasmine flowers sweeten the spirit of the target.

Saffron (cool)

Saffron is another biblical herb; it is worked with in all sweetening works.

Attraction Works

Gravelroot (cool)

Gravelroot is worked with when you are seeking a raise at work and are asking for better benefits. It is also good to add a pinch to any conjure bag that is made for finding a new job.

Orange Peel (cool)

Orange peel is worked in anything concerning drawing in our attraction work. This is one of the main ingredients in attraction products and road-opening products.

Sarsaparilla Root (dual)

Sarsaparilla root is worked for a peaceful home, prosperity, and to draw good health into the home.

These are just a small sampling of roots and herbs that can help you reach your goal in a work. This is not a complete list, but I hope it is enough to help you understand how to choose the roots and herbs for a particular work. It's always a good idea to check ingredients with your pendulum to make sure you have everything you need for the job at hand.

Checking Ingredients with a Pendulum

For those who don't know about working with the pendulum to find out if the work and ingredients are enough for success, I'll explain. As a young worker I was taught to check my work with a pendulum made from a cotton string tied on a ring. It is very important that you check your ingredients to make sure the combination of ingredients will work well together and be strong enough for success along with your prayers and petitions. If you don't learn anything else from this book, you need to remember this.

I always call on the Holy Trinity and the ancestors before I start gathering up supplies. I petition them for their help in finding the right ingredients to do the work. Then I listen. I make a list of what I think I may need. I lay out the ingredients on the list and go through them one by one with my pendulum. It takes a little while, but it is well worth it. There have been times when I simply needed a rock, moss, and dirt to do a job. It really all depends on how well you listen and how connected you are with the ancestors of this work.

The more you do the work, the more comfortable you will become with the work and finding your ingredients. It might not always be just roots and herbs—you may feel drawn to add something different; something that may seem odd. Just do the work to the best of your ability.

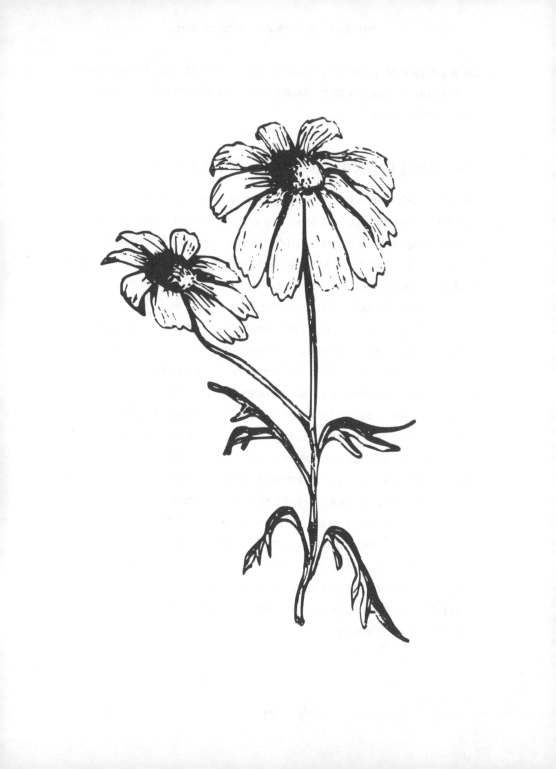

CONJURE HERBS
AND THEIR USES

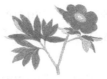

I've seen a few folks say that there are plenty of herbals out there and who needs another one? That may be true, but there isn't one like this. This section is filled with information on each herb, and you will be able to find out if the herb is hot or cold. That makes a difference in the success of your work. As far as I know, this is the first herbal that shares this information with the reader.

It is important to know what herbs are hot or cool, and some herbs have a dual purpose so they can be worked for hot or cold work. If you are trying to do a peaceful home work, you wouldn't want to add herbs that tend to be hot because they would only enflame the situation more. The same reasoning applies to love work or enemy work: you wouldn't add herbs that cool things off because you want the energy of the heat so the work can do its job.

In addition, the information here leads you into the Southern culture that this work comes from and the wisdom of the elders who have passed this work down through the generation. Roots and herbs play a large part in Conjure: they are worked for everything from powders for laying tricks to a conjure bag for prosperity. Just remember to treat them with respect: they are living beings.

You will find recipes scattered all through this herbal list. They are time-honored recipes that have shown their success time after time.

Abrus Seeds (hot)

Also called *Abrus precatorius*, known commonly as jequirity, crab's eye, rosary pea, precatory pea or bean, John Crow bead, Indian licorice, or Jumbic bead.

First off, these seeds are poisonous and should never be ingested. Abrus seeds are small and red and black. They are carried for protection and good luck.

Acacia (hot)

According to the Bible this wood was used to make the altars in the tabernacles. This is a holy wood, and it can be worked for all types of protection works.

Adam-and-Eve Roots (hot)

Adam-and-eve roots are worked with in all types of love and marriage works. The Adam root is named for the male in the relationship, and the Eve root is named for the female in the relationship. Nowadays it's hard to find the real roots. Folks are selling buds that favor the roots, but some say these buds still work.

If you are trying to get a proposal or trying to keep a lover home, you can make a conjure bag. Into this bag you would add an adam-and-eve root named for the couple. Then you can add some calamus, lovage, a magnet, and damiana root.

Calamus is worked with to be in control.

Lovage draws love and self-love.

The magnet puts strength into the draw.

Damiana is worked in all types of love works.

Adder's-Tongue (hot)

Like alum, adder's-tongue stops gossip in shut your mouth works. Adder's-tongue is good for stopping folks who try to stick their nose in your business; it even helps stop unknown backbiters. It is a good herb to add to any type of shut your mouth work.

Agrimony (hot)

Agrimony is one of my favorite herbs. It can be worked with for protection, breaking up cross conditions, and all better business and prosperity works. When added to herbs like angelica root, rue, bay leaves, and olive leaf, it makes a strong protection packet.

Alfalfa (dual)

Alfalfa is one of my favorite herbs to work with in all manner of money works. Alfalfa is also good when you are trying to protect your business or your money. I like to make a money-drawing floor sweep. You will find that some herbs do more than one thing. I called these all-purpose herbs. To make a money-drawing floor sweep, you need cornmeal, a pinch of sugar, alfalfa, orange peel, dirt from your front and back door stoop, and devil's bit.

Add all your ingredients in a glass bowl, and as you put in each ingredient, pray over it. I like to pray Psalm 23 over this type of work. Once you have the ingredients all mixed up, place you a candle in the center of the ingredients. Light your candle and pray your petition. Let the candle burn out, and then your floor sweep is ready to work with.

Alkanet Root (hot)

Alkanet root is worked with for all kinds of money works from good fortune to good business. This is the perfect root for all your prosperity needs; it also helps protect against cross conditions. The root is also good for coloring fast luck oils red. Here's a little recipe so you can make your own red fast luck oil.

Base oil

Shredded money

Alkanet root

Orange peel

Devil's bit

Add all your dry ingredients to a mason jar, and then cover the roots and herbs with your base oil. Place the jar in a crossroads candle setup, then say your prayers and your petition to be lucky in all things.

Allheal, aka Self-Heal (cool)

Allheal is worked with for all-around healing and to keep sickness away. Allheal can be placed in a white handkerchief along with three bay leaves, frankincense, three devil's shoestrings to hobble the devil, and the dirt from the front and back door of the house. Place all the ingredients in the center of the white handkerchief and call on the Trinity to drive away all illnesses from the folks in the house and from the house. Gather the hankie from corner to corner and make a knot, then gather the other two corners and make another knot. Feed the packet some whiskey and then place it either under the sickbed or beside the sickbed. After the person gets well, bury the packet in the west.

Allspice (hot)

Allspice is another great herb for money drawing and better business. You can make a floor sweep out of it. You need cornmeal, allspice, shredded money, and angelica root. Mix all your ingredients together while praying that your money be protected and drawn into your home or business. Start at the front door and sprinkle your floor sweep through the house or business. Then take your broom and sweep it to the back of the house. You can then sweep the ingredients into a clean dustpan and sprinkle them outside your door stoop or at the end of your walkway.

Aloes (hot)

Aloes is a bitter herb that is worked with to shut folk's mouths when they can't seem to mind their own business. This herb is good for all types of works concerning gossip, two-faced folks, and liars.

Althaea Leaves (cool)

Althaea leaves can be worked with to draw good spirits into a home or business. It is also wonderful as a healing herb because, like lavender, it soothes the spirit. Some folks even add it to their psychic vision oil as it is said to help increase one's psychic ability. This is one of those herbs that can be worked with for more than one condition.

Alum (hot)

Alum is another bitter herb worked with to stop gossip, but it is also worked with to remove crossed conditions. If you feel that someone has put the roots on you; you can place a chunk of alum in a cast-iron skillet and burn it over a low fire. Stir the alum with a stick from a weeping willow tree. This will remove the cross conditions, and the person who has crossed you up will weep.

Angelica (hot)

Angelica, or the Holy Ghost root as some call it, is worked with in all protection work. It is also powerful when one is dealing with family matters and unruly children. Old folks say that angelica root is the root of the angels. They say that this root is a powerful healing root. They say that when the root is petitioned for healing that it destroys anything sent to make the person ill. This is a root that everyone should keep on hand. You can add angelica root, three devil's shoe-string, and three bay leaves to a white handkerchief. Then roll the handkerchief toward you and tie it into three knots. Feed the packet some whiskey, hold it up to your mouth and say your prayer and petition into it, then hang it above your front door. The old folks say this packet will keep the devil out.

Anise Seed (cool)

Anise seeds are well known for their use in psychic vision oils and also for their ability to ward off the evil eye.

Arrowroot (hot)

Arrowroot is powdered, and some folks make sachet powders using this root as the base instead of talc. Some say that arrowroot when powdered draws good luck and money on its own.

Asafoetida (hot)

Asafoetida stinks plain and simple, but it is wonderful in run devil run works, for cross conditions, and it is even said to help keep diseases away. Old folks say that it smells so bad that even the devil can't stand it and will run away. That's why it's good in run devil run works.

Balm of Gilead (cool)

Like lavender, this is a soothing herb. It is also biblical herb. It is said to heal hurt feelings and a broken heart. It is good when you are trying to do a cut and clear. By adding it to the work, you will be settled down enough so you can truly think about the situation and the work that is at hand.

Barberry (hot)

Barberry is worked with to stop your enemies. You can mix barberry, the dirt from a stop sign, a pinch of dirt from the four corners of a crossroads that your enemy will be passing through, and a photo of your enemy burnt to ash. Place all the ingredients in a small jar and add a half a cup of milk. Close the jar and set it in the center of a crossroads candle setup with one tealight burning on top. Let the setup burn out, and then shake the jar while calling the target's name and praying your petition. Work the jar as long as you need to. Then when the work is finished, throw the jar in running water.

Basil (dual)

Basil is worked for all money matters. Basil is also good for sending evil away. It is a helpful herb to add to all run devil run works. It is also said to strengthen the love and happiness within the home. Basil is good for protection as well. Get a bundle of fresh basil and hang it inside your front door. As it dries, you can work with it as a broom and brush yourself off daily.

Bay Leaf (hot)

Bay leaf is one of Mama Starr's favorite herbs used for protection and sending the devil running. A bay leaf placed in the corner of each room and behind a photo facing the door will help protect the home. A wash of lavender, bay leaf, basil, and cinnamon can be made to wash down all the doors in the home and to clean the stoop off.

This will provide a peaceful home that is well protected and draw in prosperity.

Bayberry (hot)

Bayberry is worked with in all money-drawing and prosperity workings. I like to add a pinch of bayberry to all my better business and money works.

Benzoin Resin (cool)

Benzoin resin is worked with to preserve and add power to all types of conjure workings. It can also be worked with to purify and clear out negativity and cross conditions.

Bergamot Orange (hot)

Bergamot is worked with for all drawing and attraction work. Bergamot also adds extra power to conjure work; it could be considered a dual herb.

Blackberry Leaves (hot)

Blackberry leaves are worked with for all reversal work. These leaves will also return the evil back to the sender.

Blue Flag (hot)

Blue flag is worked with for prosperity work. It also adds extra power and protection to conjure work.

Bloodroot (hot)

Bloodroot is for all types of work dealing with the family. It can be added to all peaceful home recipes to help draw peace to the family and the home.

Bloodleaf (hot)

Bloodleaf is worked with to remove folks that you want out of your life. When mixed with salt and sulfur, it can even keep out evil spirits.

Borage Flowers (cool)

Borage flowers are worked with in all types of peaceful home workings. They are believed to calm hotheads and to bring peace to the target.

Broomstraw (dual)

Broomstraw is worked with for protection and cleansing. The old folks say that it will sweep away evil and witches. It can also be worked for crossing and jinxing.

Buckeye Nut (dual)

Buckeye nut is worked with in healing works to help with headaches, arthritis, and tied natures. It is also said to be very lucky when carried in one's pocket.

Burdock Root (dual)

Burdock root is worked with for all cleansing and uncrossing work. It is also said to restore a male condition that has been jinxed.

Calendula Flowers (dual)

Calendula flowers are worked in court case works. They are also very good in healing salves or for making warm compresses for achy muscles.

Calamus (hot)

Calamus helps for all domination work. Calamus is also good to add to all types of protection work.

Capsicum spp

Red pepper is worked with to heat things up when you are doing a job. It will heat the target's head up, and unless you are doing a crossing work, it shouldn't be added. It is one of the ingredients in Hotfoot Powder.

Caraway Seed (hot)

Caraway seeds are good to have with all types of protection work. You can tie caraway seeds, angelica root, and three bay leaves in a white handkerchief, and then hang the handkerchief over a child's bed to keep nightmares away.

Cardamom Seed (hot)

Cardamom seeds are worked with to bring forth heat and lust in a relationship. It is also said that they will make the wearer lucky in love.

Cascara Sagrada (hot)

Cascara sagrada is worked with when you have a tough court case. It is also said to bring good luck.

Catnip (cool)

Catnip is worked with when a woman wants to draw her man really close. It is a good herb to add to any follow me boy work.

Cayenne Pepper (hot)

Cayenne pepper is good in all hot foot work and all enemy work. It is also worked with when you need to heat a work up—in other words when you need to add some fire to the work. You need to be careful when working with cayenne pepper because it is so hot.

Cedarwood (hot)

Cedar is worked with for protection and also for rotting a relationship. Have you ever noticed how a cedar tree always rots from the inside out? Take a photo of the target and bury it under a cedar tree as close to the trunk as you can get. As the tree rots so will the relationship.

Celandine (hot)

Celandine is worked with in confusing work, especially for court cases. It is also good to add to any loss stay away products.

Celery Seed (hot)

Celery seeds are added to psychic vision oil to help bring forth dreams that are clear and show what the worker is trying to find out.

Chamomile Flowers or Manzanilla (cool)

Chamomile flowers are worked with for uncrossing and protection. They are also added to lucky hands and washes. Chamomile is very good when made into a tea to soothe a nervous stomach or a restless spirit.

Chia Seed (hot)

Chia seeds can be added to all types of works that deal with gossip, backbiting, and two-faced folks. Mix a pinch of chia seeds with red pepper and alum to shut the backbiters up.

Cinnamon (hot)

Cinnamon is added to all types of work where money and luck are needed in a hurry. It is also one of the herbs that are added to the recipe of holy oil that comes right out of the Bible. So it's safe to say it is also worked with for blessings and protection work.

Clover Flowers, Red (hot)

Red clover flowers are worked with in all marriage and love works. The old folks say that they bring forth a lucky and prosperous marriage.

Clover Flowers, White (cool)

White clover flowers are worked with in all works for cleansing and purification. It is said that white clover will drive away all evil.

Cloves (hot)

Cloves are worked with in some shut your mouth work, but they are well known for the power they bring to all conjure works for prosperity and better business.

Coriander Seed (dual)

Coriander seeds can be worked with as an offering for Moses. It is also said that they are good for keeping passion in a relationship and your mate faithful.

Coltsfoot (cool)

Coltsfoot can be added to a spiritual wash to remove illness from a sickroom. It is also said that it can be mixed with other herbs to bring forth psychic visions.

Comfrey (cool)

Comfrey helps you hold on to the money you have or the money that you win while gambling. It is good for safety when you are away from home.

Couch Grass (hot)

Couch grass can bind your enemies and is also worked in some love Conjure.

Cubeb Berries (hot)

Cubeb berries can be added to attraction work to draw a new person into your life. It is also said that it can be added to other roots and herbs to get control of your mate.

Cumin Seed (hot)

Cumin seeds come right out of the Bible. They are worked with when you need to deflect evil and cut away bad luck. They can be added to a wash or a conjure bag.

Damiana (hot)

It is said that damiana is the number one love herb that should be added to all love works. I work with it and some love works, but I prefer lovage.

Dandelion Root (cool)

Dandelion root is worked with to help you gain the second sight. It can be carried in a conjure bag along with celery seed, bay leaf, and frankincense.

Deer's-Tongue (dual)

Deer's-tongue can be worked with when you have a court case; it also helps you charm the judge. Deer's-tongue added to a love work helps insure a ring on the finger.

Devil's Bit (hot)

Devil's bit holds the devil down and is worked with in all uncrossing and protection workings. Devil's bit is one of the main ingredients in the run devil run products.

Devil Pod (hot)

Devil pod provides strong protection against evil and any dark spirits sent by an enemy to harm you. Get a small devil pod, feed it whiskey, then place it in a candle setup. Once the candles burn out, place the devil pod in a red flannel bag and carry it at your waist, or if you're a woman, you can carry it in your bosom.

Devil's Shoestring (hot)

Devil's shoestring is worked with in all enemy work. Three devil's shoestrings tied together with your photo in the center of them is strong protection and will send the devil running. Devil's shoestrings are also worked in all work to nail the devil down.

Dill (hot)

Dill is a sour herb, so therefore, it is worked with in all types of souring work.

Dixie John Root (hot)

Dixie John root is worked for protection, luck, and also to keep a spouse faithful. When combined with the other John roots—High John the Conqueror and Little John—it makes a powerful conjure bag that makes the wearer almost undefeatable.

Dragon's Blood (hot)

Dragon's blood keeps evil away and brings spiritual empowerment to the user.

Elderflowers (dual)

Elderflowers are worked with in all matter of protection work—even protection from the law.

Eucalyptus (cool)

Eucalyptus is worked with in all types of cleansing work; it is also said that it will drive spirits out of the home. If you sprinkle eucalyptus leaves across the doorway when an enemy leaves, they won't be back. The trick is that they walk over the leaves when they leave the house.

Eyebright (cool)

Eyebright is a healing herb first and foremost. If you are having issues with your eyes, a cool bath of eyebright will help soothe them. Eyebright is also worked with in Conjure to see what is hidden and also to help the workers see a situation clearly.

Fennel Seed (hot)

Fennel seeds are worked with to keep away all types of government folks.

Fenugreek Seed (hot)

Mama Starr loves this stuff! It is worked for drawing money and luck into your home. Add fenugreek seeds to a small white bowl with a pinch of sugar and some shredded money. Place this high in the kitchen on top of the icebox. This is a trick Mama Starr works to keep prosperity coming into her home.

Fern (cool)

Fern is worked with for protection, love, and to remove crossed conditions by brushing yourself down with three fern leaves.

Feverfew (cool)

Feverfew is worked with as a wash. It is added to a tub of cool water to relieve a fever. It is also added to protection packets for folks who tend to always end up being harmed or hurt in accidents.

Five Finger Grass (dual)

Five finger grass is worked with for luck, love, money, and protection. The old folks say that five finger grass can do anything that the five fingers on the hand can do. So this is a very good ingredient for all types of work when you are trying to draw something to you.

Flaxseed (dual)

Flaxseed is worked for all issues concerning the home and protection; it is also a good conjure herb for the second sight.

Frankincense Resin (dual)

Frankincense is a tree resin mentioned in the Bible. This is one of the most holy gifts that the wise men brought to baby Jesus. It is said that it is a powerful tool for spiritual protection. It also adds power to any type of work.

Garlic (hot)

Garlic is another herb right out of the Bible. It is worked with to remove all types of evil spirits and is powerful for protection in conjure work.

Ginseng Root (hot)

Ginseng root is worked with in all types of money and gambling jobs. It is a very hot root, so it can heat up all types of work. It is also said to enhance the male vigor.

Goldenseal Root (cool)

Goldenseal root is used in all types of work where wisdom is needed. It is also said that it lends strength to the worker.

Grains of Paradise (hot)

Grains of paradise are worked with for all types of protection, money, and steady work jobs and are also said to make wishes come true. You can add grains of paradise to any conjure work to heat the work up.

Gravelroot (cool)

Gravelroot is worked with when you are seeking a raise or asking for better benefits at your job. It is also good to add a pinch to any conjure bag that is made for finding a new job.

Hawthorn Berries (hot)

Hawthorn berries are very protective. They are added to conjure bags or packets for extra protection. You can make a tea out of them and wash your front and back door with it to protect your home.

High John the Conqueror (hot)

High John the Conqueror is worked with in all types of blockbuster work. It is said that there is not a block in the world that this root can't get through. It is also very good for helping with personal power and self-esteem.

Holly Leaves (hot)

Holly leaves are very protective. The tree is also worked with for protection, and in some places you will see one planted on each side of the door.

Honeysuckle (cool)

Honeysuckle is worked with in all types of sweetening works. A honeysuckle vine can be wrapped around a photo of you and your lover to draw you closer together and to sweeten the love you have for each other.

Hops (cool)

Hops are worked with for peaceful sleep and to keep nightmares away. Get a white handkerchief, a pinch of hops, a pinch of lavender, and three bay leaves named after God the Father, God the Son, and God the Holy Spirit. Place all the ingredients in the handkerchief and tie three knots in it in the name of the Trinity. Place the handkerchief inside your pillow. This will help you have a peaceful night's sleep.

Hyssop (cool)

Hyssop is worked with in all types of protection, run devil run, and jinx-removing works. Hyssop is another powerful herb right out of the Bible. It is also said to add power to all types of conjure work.

Irish Moss (dual)

Irish moss is worked with to draw prosperity and also for protection. Irish moss can also be employed in all types of crossing work; that is one of the reasons that it is a dual herb.

Jalapeño (hot)

Jalapeños are worked with to heat up all types of enemy work, from shut your mouth to run devil run.

Jasmine Flowers (cool)

Jasmine flowers are worked with in all types of love works. It is also said that jasmine flowers sweeten the spirit of the target.

Jezebel Root (hot)

Jezebel root is worked with for all domination work. It is also said that it gives power and self-esteem to women. This root is a woman's root and keeps the woman in total control of her life.

Job's Tears (dual)

Job's tears are very powerful. Seven seeds worked for seven days are said to grant an important wish. The old folks will tell you that Job's tears can be worked to make an enemy shed as many tears as Job did.

Juniper Berries (hot)

Juniper berries attract love. It is said that when a woman carries them in a packet, they will draw a lover to her.

Knotweed (hot)

Knotweed is worked with for all binding and blocking works. It can also be worked with in bend over, domination, and control workings.

Lavender (cool)

Lavender brings a peaceful home. Lavender soothes and cools down the spirit. It works wonders for folks who are hotheaded and bullheaded.

Lemon Leaves (cool)

Lemon leaves are worked with in all cut and clear works, which also includes road-opening works. Cut and clear work is not just to cut old love out of your life; it can also remove all things holding you back.

Lemongrass (cool)

Lemongrass is worked in all jinx-removing and uncrossing works. It is one of the main ingredients in Van Van oil.

Lemon Mint (dual)

Lemon mint breaks up old conditions. It is added to some road-opening works.

Lemon Verbena (cool)

Lemon verbena is worked with for breakup works. It is said to cause fussing and fighting to tear the targets apart from each other.

Life Everlasting (cool)

It is said that this herb promotes a longer life; it can be added to all healing works. Brew it into an herbal tea and drink daily for longer life.

Little John (hot)

Chewing Little John adds to your personal power. When you join this John with the other two Johns—High John the Conqueror and Dixie John—it is unbeatable. It is famous for court case works.

Licorice Root (hot)

Licorice root comes in handy in all domination workings. It also generally adds power and strength to conjure work.

Lovage (dual)

Lovage is worked with in all love works. It is particularly wonderful when you are working on yourself; it promotes self-love and a high self-esteem. In washes or sprinkled around the home, it brings love and peace to the place.

Mandrake (dual)

Mandrake is another of the biblical herbs. It is worked with when dealing with love issues and also to draw money in.

Marjoram (hot)

Marjoram is worked with to drive off those folks who would harm your family. It is also worked with to protect a home or business from jinxes.

Master of the Woods (hot)

Master of the Woods is worked with in all domination and commanding work.

Master Root (hot)

Master root is worked with licorice root, calamus, and Master of the Woods for the mastering of power in any situation.

Mint (hot)

Mint is another biblical herb. It is worked for breaking jinxes and to run the devil off.

Mojo Beans (cool)

Mojo beans, also known as wishing beans or fava beans, are worked with in all money and luck work.

Motherwort (cool)

Motherwort is worked with in all efforts concerning your children. It is also good for all family and protection work dealing with women and children.

Mugwort (dual)

Mugwort can open up the psychic connection to reach the spirit world. It improves the intuition.

Mullein (hot)

Mullein is worked with to draw in spirits. It is also worked with in the dark arts.

Mustard Seeds, Black (hot)

Black mustard seeds can cause confusion and loss of concentration when a target is being worked on. The target will have had a time focusing on their job and life in general.

Mustard Seeds, White (hot)

White mustard seeds are another herb from the Bible, as in "Job had the faith of a mustard seed." They are good to work with in all protection work and works of faith.

Myrrh (dual)

Myrrh is a tree resin mentioned in the Bible that is worked with for protection and to add extra power in all conjure working.

Nettles (hot)

Nettles are worked with for uncrossing and jinx breaking works. Nettles can also be a crossing herb because of the stings.

Nutmeg (hot)

Nutmeg is worked with in all money matters, all dealings with prosperity work, and anything to do with drawing good fortune into your life.

Oak (cool)

Oak is worked with to add personal power to any work and also helps with cleansing works to remove jinxed and cross conditions.

Orange Peel (cool)

Orange peel is helpful concerning anything that is drawing or attracting. This is one of the main ingredients in attraction products and road-opening products.

Oregano (hot)

Oregano is worked with in all matters dealing with the law, whether that is law stay away or to keep troublesome folks away.

Passionflower (cool)

Passionflower is worked with in all peace and blessing work. Passionflower is said to bring forth love.

Patchouli (hot)

Patchouli can be worked with in all love-drawing, domination, crossing, money-drawing, and uncrossing works.

Pennyroyal (cool)

Pennyroyal can cool heads and keep peace in a home. It is worked with to stop family arguments and to help heal marriage problems.

Peony Root (dual)

Peony root is worked with to break old jinxes and to draw forth good fortune. It is said to help the wearer against misfortune. It can also be worked to bring misfortune on a target.

Pepper, Black (hot)

Black pepper is worked with in some move out workings. I personally prefer red pepper because it's hotter. Black pepper will also remove fussing and fighting in a home.

Periwinkle (dual)

Periwinkle is carried to help ward off the evil eye. It can also be placed under your mattress on the side of the target to help in all matters of love. You can carry a little in your wallet to help attract more money.

Pine Tree Resin (hot)

Pine tree resin is useful for some controlling works, but it can also be worked when you want to nail down a job. Pine resin is also good in healing works: it was employed in the old days to seal cuts and scrapes.

Poppy Seeds (hot)

Poppy seeds are worked with to cause confusion and delays in all enemy works. It is also worked with to cause your enemy to weaken and to dominate them. Some say it can help with psychic visions and dreams when you're asleep.

Quassia (hot)

Quassia is worked with in all shut your mouth works or works concerning controlling and dominating a target.

Queen Elizabeth Root (dual)

Queen Elizabeth root is worked with by women to draw power, love, and luck with the opposite sex. It also adds to a woman's personal power and her self-esteem.

Raspberry Leaves (hot)

Raspberry leaves help women keep their men at home and stop them from rambling. It can be placed in a conjure bag or a spiritual bath along with other roots and herbs that focus on keeping your man faithful.

Rattlesnake Master (hot)

Rattlesnake master is worked with to keep them snakes in the grass under control. It helps with protection against hidden enemies and known enemies.

Rosebuds (hot)

Rosebuds are worked with in all love-drawing works to promote love.

Rose Petals (hot)

Rose petals are worked with in all love and romance situations. Rose petals are also a wonderful offering for Mother Mary.

Rosemary (dual)

Rosemary is added to all works done by women because this is a woman's herb that gives women extra power and puts them in charge of their homes and environments. It can also be worked with in all protection works and in spiritual cleansings. It will remove all crossed conditions.

Rue (dual)

Rue is worked with to remove all crossed conditions. It gives the worker power to help find and destroy all enemies known and unknown. It is a good herb to add to fiery wall of protection products.

Saffron (cool)

Saffron is another biblical herb; it is worked with in all sweetening works.

Sage (cool)

Sage is burnt to clear out an area. It also brings forth blessings and helps with wisdom and the common sense to find the answers that one is seeking.

Sampson Snakeroot (hot)

Sampson snakeroot is worked with to add power and strength to any works. It is mostly worked with by men.

Sarsaparilla Root (dual)

Sarsaparilla root is worked with for peaceful home, prosperity, and to draw good health into the home.

Sassafras Root (dual)

Sassafras root is worked with for all money, prosperity, and success works. Sassafras oil is also good for the treatment of head and body lice.

Self Heal (cool)

Self heal is worked with in all health matters and is said to help cleanse and heal the sick.

Seneca Snakeroot (hot)

Seneca snakeroot, also known as rattlesnake root, is worked with to keep those snake-in-the-grass two-faced liars away from you. It is said to protect the wearer against liars and false friends.

Senna Leaf (dual)

Senna leaf is worked with to attract a new person who is not aware of your interest and also helps in all reconciliation and love works to keep your partner faithful.

Slippery Elm (hot)

Slippery elm is worked with when you want to hide yourself and the work that you are doing from your enemy. It also hides you from your enemies who are trying to work on you. Be cautious with this herb: a little bit goes a long way.

Solomon's Seal Root (cool)

Named for King Solomon of the Bible, this root is for wisdom, power, and protection in all conjure works.

Spanish Moss (dual)

For good or evil conjure workings, Spanish moss can be used to protect your home or draw money but is also very useful for crossing work.

Spikenard (dual)

Spikenard is another biblical herb used for love workings. Spikenard is good to add to your love works along with a pinch of Master of the Woods.

Star Anise (dual)

For protection, good luck, prosperity, and healing works, star anise is also said to help with psychic power.

Tansy (cool)

Tansy is worked with for protection against the police, DEA, or INS. It is said to keep these government officials from looking into one's affairs.

Ten Bark (cool)

Ten bark is worked with to help clear away the effects of an unnatural illness caused by crossed condition or being hexed by an enemy.

Thyme (dual)

Thyme is good for all money and prosperity works. It is also good for cleansing and protection works. You can make a wash out of a pinch of thyme, three bay leaves, and some rue. Wash down your doors and then take a spiritual bath in some of the wash.

Tobacco (hot)

You can work with tobacco leaf to bind and hold an enemy down. Tobacco is also good for feeding Spirit and drawing spirits to an altar.

Tonka Bean (cool)

Tonka beans are good for all workings of love and luck. The old folks say that it is really lucky if you carry three tonka beans tied up in a white handkerchief and fed whiskey once a week. Carry the packet in your pocket or bosom for good luck.

Vandalroot (hot)

Vandalroot is worked with for causing crossed conditions against an enemy. It is also said to be used for making pacts and drawing dark spirits.

Verbena (hot)

Verbena is a love-drawing herb and is worked with in all love works.

Violet Leaf (cool)

Violet leaves can be worked with when you have a broken heart. They are also said to help draw back a lost love. Violet leaves can be added to works when you are trying to draw a new love.

Walnut (dual)

Walnuts are worked with for jinxing and uncrossing a target. They may also be worked with for breakup.

Willow (hot)

Willow is worked with to remove cross conditions and jinxes, but it is also good to put on cross conditions and jinxes.

Wintergreen (hot)

Wintergreen is worked with to draw prosperity, money, and good money. It can be burned as an incense or sprinkled across the door stoop to draw in prosperity and money.

Wood Betony (dual)

Wood betony is worked with to keep away evil spirits and to reverse crossed conditions.

Wormwood (dual)

Wormwood is worked with to prevent accidents, and when added to protection work, it's a powerful ally. It can also be worked with to help contact spirits.

Yarrow Flower (dual)

Yarrow flowers are worked with when you need the courage to do something. They also help improve psychic powers and are said to break up crossed conditions.

CONJURE OILS
AND THEIR USES

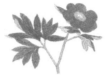

C onjure oils are made by combining a base oil with herbs and other conjure materials. In this section of the book I want to share some information about conjure oils and how to work with them. And I want to share five of my recipes so you can make your own oils. A lot of folks who sell these products get upset with me because I give too much information away in my books, but the thing is these things need to be shared so they can live on.

Every oil starts with some type of base oil. In the old days when I was coming up, olive oil, castor oil, sweet oil, mineral oil, and lard were what was worked with because that is what folks had on hand. Below are some base oils that can be blended into conjure oils.

Base Oils

Almond oil

Castor oil

Coconut oil

Grapeseed oil

Jojoba oil

Mineral oil

Sunflower seed oil

Sweet oil

Olive oil is a most holy oil. It is found all through God's word, as in these examples.

> *Isaiah 61 V 3*
>
> *To appoint unto them that mourn in Zion, to give unto them beauty for ashes, the oil of joy for mourning, the garment of praise for the spirit of heaviness; that they might be called trees of righteousness, the planting of the Lord, that he might be glorified.*
>
> *Exodus 29 V 7*
>
> *Then shalt thou take the anointing oil, and pour it upon his head, and anoint him.*
>
> *1 Kings 17 V 12*
>
> *But she said, "As the Lord your God lives, I have no bread, only a handful of flour in the bowl and a little oil in the jar; and behold, I am*

*gathering a few sticks that I may go in and
prepare for me and my son, that we may eat it
and die."*

Leviticus 24 V 2

*Command the children of Israel, that they bring
unto thee pure oil olive beaten for the light, to
cause the lamps to burn continually.*

Leviticus 2 V 15

*You shall then put oil on it and lay incense on it;
it is a grain offering.*

Conjure Oils in General and Their Uses

Attraction Oil

Attraction oil is used for attracting financial blessing, romance, good luck, and success. You can use this oil to dress your money and yourself to aid in drawing in your desires.

Blackhawk Oil

Blackhawk oil is a very special oil of empowerment in honor of the great chief Blackhawk of the Sauk Nation. When used, his spirit and power give you a helping hand in your conjure work. This oil also aids in connecting to other Native ancestral spirits.

Crown of Success Oil

Crown of success is a popular conjure oil traditionally used to empower positive results in business, money, and schooling. It is also said to aid in helping a person go the distance and achieve limitless success in all ventures.

Cut and Remove Oil

This is an old conjure favorite. This special oil is formulated to aid in letting go negative people and the past. It helps to remove unrequited loves and old flames from your life so that you can move on.

Fiery Wall of Protection Oil

One of the strongest of the conjure oils, Fiery Wall of Protection builds a wall of security around an individual and their loved one and safeguards them from their enemies.

Hotfoot Oil

If there are unwanted people you need out of your life, this is the oil to use.

Master Key Oil

Powerful Master Key oil is used to achieve success and unlock doorways of possibility.

Run Devil Run Oil

This spiritual oil of protection and banishment is used against the devil and all his tricks. Also used for luck, love, and money conjure works.

Uncrossing Oil

This oil works to remove all setbacks, roadblocks, and crossed conditions.

Van Van Oil

One of the oldest and most powerful oils in Conjure, Van Van oil is used for protection, clearing evil, and adding power to conjure bags, amulets, altars, and general rootworking needs.

Oil Recipes

Blood of Jesus Oil

The blood of Jesus is the most powerful blood you can call on. Pray the Sacred Heart of Jesus Prayer over the ingredients of your oil. Then add all the ingredients into the olive oil and pray over it again. Set the oil in a cross setup of red candles, and then pray the Sacred Heart of Jesus Prayer over the oil three times a day until the candles burn out.

Sacred Heart of Jesus Prayer

> *O most holy heart of Jesus, fountain of every blessing. I adore you, I love you, and with lively sorrow for my sins, I offer you this poor heart of mine. Make me humble, patient, pure, and wholly obedient to your will. Grant, Good Jesus, that I may live in you and for you. Protect me in the midst of danger. Comfort me in my afflictions. Give me health of body, assistance in my temporal needs, your blessing on all that I do, and the grace of a holy death. Amen.*

Olive oil base (biblical holy oil)

Angelica root (Holy Ghost root)

Devil's shoestring (to hobble the devil)

Frankincense (biblical resin of protection)

Myrrh (biblical resin of cleansing)

Hyssop (biblical herb for protection and cleansing)

Barberry (holy thorn herb against enemies)

Mama Starr's Special All-Around Conjure Oil

Master of the Woods (for power)

Orange peel (for attraction)

Angelica (for blessings)

Devil's shoestring (to hobble the devil)

Shut Your Mouth Conjure Oil

Alum (to sour)

Dirt dauber (for power)

Dried red peppers (to heat)

Self-Love Conjure Oil

Lovage root (to promote love)

Angelica root (for blessings)

Bloodroot (to draw love)

Money Draw Conjure Oil

A piece of magnet (to draw)

Five finger grass (to grab)

Angelica root (for blessings)

Psalm 23

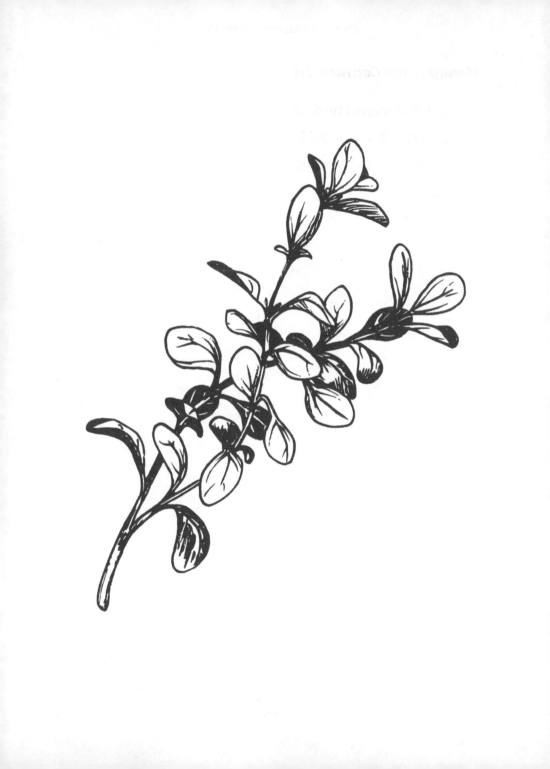

CONJURE RECIPES AND WORKINGS WITH HERBS, ROOTS, AND OILS

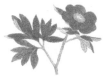

T he one thing that you need to remember is that herbs, roots, and oils are just those raw materials until you add prayer to them. It's only then that they become a workable product. You can just throw something together and hope for the best, or you can put your products in a candle setup and pray over them daily for at least five days to have a powerful tool. Everyone knows that prayer brings the power.

You can work with the basic cross setup to empower your recipes. The way you do this is place the tealights one at the top, one at the bottom, one to the right, and one to the left. Then set your product in the center and light your candles in the same order you set them down. Say your prayer over your product. Repeat this method at least once a day for five days.

The recipes I am sharing here will help you get an idea of how to work your own. The oil recipe will come first, and it should be assumed that candles in the works that follow should be dressed with it.

Recipes for Money

Money Oil

> Bayberry
>
> Magnetic sand
>
> Calamus root

To Draw Money

For this work you will be using a stick candle. Burn your petition to ash and mix with powdered herbs. You can use just cinnamon and sugar if that is all you have. Write your name on the candle, then dress the candle toward you with oil (from top to bottom). Roll the candle in your powder *toward* you. Holding the candle close to your mouth, say your prayer, then light your stick candle and place it in a candleholder. When the candle burns out, bury any leftover wax in your yard in the east. Repeat this process for five days when the hands of the clock are moving upward.

Blockbuster Candle

In this work you will use a large pillar candle. If you can find an orange one, then use orange. But if you can't, then use a white one. Take a pair of small scissors or a knife and dig a hole either in the bottom or the side of the candle. (The reason you use scissors or a knife is because you are removing the blocks that are holding you back.) Save the wax from the hole. You need a plate to set your candle on. You will also need John 14 V 1-14 torn from an old Bible, your petition paper, and one small piece of High John root. Burn the Bible verse to ash along with your petition; mix this with a little powdered angelica root. Load your powder and the High John into the hole. Fill the hole with the wax you removed. Write your name on the candle along with "I knocked and the door was opened." Set the candle on the plate and sprinkle the leftover powder around the candle. Light the candle and pray for all blocks to be removed. Once the candle has burned out, take any leftover wax to the crossroads along with five pennies and leave them there.

Attraction Stick Candle

Get a red stick candle for this work. You need a large flat magnet, a round mirror, and a can. You need a picture of your desire. Write your name in the wax. Then over your name write "the Lord is my Shepherd, I shall not want." It doesn't matter if you can read what you have written. That is not the important part—the words are. Burn your petition to ash, then mix a pinch of attraction powder with the ash and mix it up well while praying your petition. Then dress your candle with a little Attraction oil, and roll it in your herbal mixture. Set your candle on the magnet. Pour a ring of sugar around the candle. Then pour a ring of whiskey over the sugar. Light the candle and say your prayers that what you are in need of will come to you. Let your candle burn until it burns out. Bury the leftovers in your yard facing the east or by your front door. Repeat this process for five days as the hands of the clock are moving upward.

Recipes for Love

Love Oil

> Lovage
>
> Lavender
>
> Queen Elizabeth root

Love Binding

This is a simple but effective binding work. Cut a small square of red flannel cloth; place Ecclesiastes 4 V 8-12 on the cloth. Take a photo of yourself and one of the target and place them face-to-face while praying Ecclesiastes 4 V 8-12 over them. Call the target's name after each verse. Place a pinch of Master of the Woods on top of the photos. Wrap all this into a small packet; bind the packet with red cotton string. Pray Ecclesiastes 4 V 8-12 as you are wrapping the string; call the target's name after each verse. Burn a tealight on it daily while praying your petition.

> *8 There is one alone, and there is not a second;*
> *yea, he hath neither child not brother: yet is there*
> *no end of all his labour; neither is his eye satis-*
> *fied with riches; neither saith he, For whom do I*
> *labour, and bereave my soul of good? This is also*
> *vanity, yea, it is a sore travail.*
>
> *9 Two are better than one; because they have a*
> *good reward for their labour.*
>
> *10 For if they fall, the one will lift up his fellow;*
> *but woe to him that is alone when he falleth; for*
> *he hath not another to help him up.*

11 Again, if two lie together, then they have heat; but how can one be warm alone?

12 And if one prevail against him, two shall withstand him; and a threefold cord is not quickly broken.

Love Drawing

You need a piece of red flannel, red string, master root, calamus, pomegranate seed, your photo, a photo of your target, and a magnet.

Place your photo and your target's photo together facing each other with the magnet between the photos. Tear out Song of Solomon 7 V 1-13 from an old Bible and wrap it around the photos and the magnet. Sprinkle your roots and herbs around the bundle and wrap red flannel around your work into a little packet. Take the red string and wrap it around your packet while saying your prayers three times. Tie three knots in the name of God the Father, God the Son, and God the Holy Ghost.

1 How beautiful are thy feet with shoes, O prince's daughter! The joints of thy thighs are like jewels, the work of the hands of a cunning workman.

2 Thy navel is like a round goblet, which wanteth not liquor: thy belly is like an heap of wheat set about with lilies.

3 Thy two breasts are like two young roes that are twins.

4 Thy neck is as a tower of ivory; thine eyes like the fishpools in Heshbon, by the gate of

Bathrabbim: thy nose is as the tower of Lebanon which looketh toward Damascus.

5 Thine head upon thee is like Carmel, and the hair of thine head like purple; the king is held in the galleries.

6 How fair and how pleasant art thou, O love, for delights!

7 This thy stature is like to a palm tree, and thy breasts to clusters of grapes.

8 I said, I will go up to the palm tree, I will take hold of the boughs thereof: now also thy breasts shall be as clusters of the vine, and the smell of thy nose like apples;

9 And the roof of thy mouth like the best wine for my beloved, that goeth down sweetly, causing the lips of those that are asleep to speak.

10 I am my beloved's, and his desire is toward me.

11 Come, my beloved, let us go forth into the field; let us lodge in the villages.

12 Let us get up early to the vineyards; let us see if the vine flourish, whether the tender grape appear, and the pomegranates bud forth: there will I give thee my loves.

13 The mandrakes give a smell, and at our gates are all manner of pleasant fruits, new and old, which I have laid up for thee, O my beloved.

Recipes for Healing

Healing Oil

> Master of the Woods
>
> Angelica
>
> Frankincense

Healing Work

Take three white candle and wipe yourself going downward with each one of them while praying Hosea 6 V 1-3 and having faith that God will heal you. Then set the candles up in a triangle setup and place your photo in the center of the setup. Pray daily for healing. Repeat as necessary.

> *1 Come, and let us return to the LORD; For He has torn, but He will heal us; He has stricken, but He will bind us up.*
>
> *2 After two days He will revive us; On the third day He will raise us up, That we may live in His sight.*
>
> *3 Let us know, Let us pursue the knowledge of the LORD. His going forth is established as the morning; He will come to us like the rain, Like the latter and former rain to the earth.*

Recipes for Blessing

Blessing Oil

> Calamus root
>
> Myrrh
>
> Bergamot

Blessing Work

When it seems that nothing is going right and like all our blessings are gone, fear not because the God of Abraham has given his word that we will not do without. Write your name in the wax of a blue candle. Dress the candle with olive oil that has been prayed over. Call on God with your need. Light the candle and pray Genesis 26 V 24 over the candle three times. Do this daily until the candle burns out. Have faith of Abraham and *know* your blessings are coming.

> *24 And the LORD appeared unto him the same night, and said, I am the God of Abraham thy father: fear not, for I am with thee, and will bless thee, and multiply thy seed for my servant Abraham's sake.*

To Draw a Blessing

Take a white bowl and place a blue candle in the center of the bowl. Write your petition on the candle. Around the candle sprinkle coriander seed, olive oil, and honey. Call on God and Moses, then light your candle. Pray Exodus 34 V 6-10 over your candle daily until the candle burns out. The blessing you need will be yours.

*6 And the LORD passed by before him, and pro-
claimed, The LORD, The LORD God, merciful
and gracious, long-suffering, and abundant in
goodness and truth,*

*7 Keeping mercy for thousands, forgiving iniq-
uity and transgression and sin, and that will by
no means clear the guilty; visiting the iniquity of
the fathers upon the children, and upon the children's children, unto the third and to the fourth
generation.*

*8 And Moses made haste, and bowed his head
toward the earth, and worshipped.*

*9 And he said, If now I have found grace in
thy sight, O LORD, let my LORD, I pray thee, go
among us; for it is a stiff-necked people; and par-
don our iniquity and our sin, and take us for
thine inheritance.*

*10 And he said, Behold, I make a covenant: before
all thy people I will do marvels, such as have not
been done in all the earth, nor in any nation: and
all the people among which thou art shall see the
work of the LORD: for it is a terrible thing that I
will do with thee.*

Blessing

To draw God's blessing, dress a blue candle with oil, and write your
name in the wax. Call on God and Moses and talk to them about
your situation. Light your candle and pray Numbers 6 V 22-27 over
your candle. Do this daily until the candle burns out.

22 And the LORD spake unto Moses, saying,

23 Speak unto Aaron and unto his sons, saying, On this wise ye shall bless the children of Israel, saying unto them,

24 The LORD bless thee, and keep thee:

25 The LORD make his face shine upon thee, and be gracious unto thee:

26 The LORD lift up his countenance upon thee, and give thee peace.

27 And they shall put my name upon the children of Israel, and I will bless them.

Recipes for Uncrossing

Uncrossing Oil

Frankincense

Bay leaves

Mint

Uncrossing Work

Write your petition and place it in the Bible in Judges 15 V 10-17, and close the Bible. Take the Bible and wipe yourself from head to toe with it while praying to God to remove any crossed condition on you. Take a white vigil candle and repeat the process. Do not dress this vigil. Light the vigil and pray Judges 15 V 10-17 over the vigil three times a day.

10 And the men of Judah said, Why are ye come up against us? And they answered, To bind Samson are we come up, to do to him as he hath done to us.

11 Then three thousand men of Judah went to the top of the rock Etam, and said to Samson, Knowest thou not that the Philistines are rulers over us? What is this that thou hast done unto us? And he said unto them, As they did unto me, so have I done unto them.

12 And they said unto him, We are come down to bind thee, that we may deliver thee into the hand of the Philistines. And Samson said unto them, Swear unto me, that ye will not fall upon me yourselves.

13 And they spake unto him, saying, No; but we will bind thee fast, and deliver thee into their hand: but surely we will not kill thee. And they bound him with two new cords, and brought him up from the rock.

14 And when he came unto Lehi, the Philistines shouted against him: and the Spirit of the LORD came mightily upon him, and the cords that were upon his arms became as flax that was burnt with fire, and his bands loosed from off his hands.

15 And he found a new jawbone of an ass, and put forth his hand, and took it, and slew a thousand men therewith.

16 And Samson said, With the jawbone of an ass, heaps upon heaps, with the jaw of an ass have I slain a thousand men.

17 And it came to pass, when he had made an end of speaking, that he cast away the jawbone out of his hand, and called that place Ramathlehi.

Recipe for Protection

Protection Oil

> Dragon's blood
>
> Devil's claw
>
> White mustard seed

Protection Work

For this work you need a red glass-encased candle. Dress the candle with protection oil. Write your petition on the candle and your name inside the candle in the wax. Tear out Genesis 19 V 6-11 from a Bible, and burn it to ash. Place the ash mixed with a drop of olive oil into the vigil candle. Light your candle and petition God for his protection. Pray Genesis 19 V 6-11 over your candle daily. Petition God to blind your enemies where they cannot find you.

> *6 And Lot went out at the door unto them, and shut the door after him,*
>
> *7 And said, I pray you, brethren, do not so wickedly.*

8 Behold now, I have two daughters which have not known man; let me, I pray you, bring them out unto you, and do ye to them as is good in your eyes: only unto these men do nothing; for therefore came they under the shadow of my roof.

9 And they said, Stand back. And they said again, this one fellow came in to sojourn, and he will needs be a judge: now will we deal worse with thee, than with them. And they pressed sore upon the man, even Lot, and came near to break the door.

10 But the men put forth their hand, and pulled Lot into the house to them, and shut to the door.

11 And they smote the men that were at the door of the house with blindness, both small and great: so that they wearied themselves to find the door.

Protection Work

There are times when we find ourselves in need of protection from someone for whatever reason. Genesis 31 V 51-52 gives us this protection. By praying this daily, there will be a pillar or a wall so to say between you and the offender. You need a white vigil. On one side write your name, on the other side write the other person's name. Dress the candle with olive oil, light the candle and pray verses Genesis 31 V 51-52 over the candle, call the person's name out after each verse. Do this daily until the vigil burns out.

51 And Laban said to Jacob, Behold this heap, and behold this pillar, which I have cast betwixt me and thee:

52 This heap be witness, and this pillar be witness, that I will not pass over this heap to thee, and that thou shalt not pass over this heap and this pillar unto me, for harm.

Protection

If you find yourself in need of protection, call on God and Moses, and petition them to protect you. Take a red candle and write your name in the wax. Dress the candle with olive oil, then light it and pray Numbers 23 V 23-24 over your candle three times. Do this daily for five days.

23 There is no divination against Jacob, no evil omens against Israel. It will now be said of Jacob and of Israel, "See what God has done!"

24 The people rise like a lioness; they rouse themselves like a lion that does not rest till it devours its prey and drinks the blood of its victims.

Recipe for Justice

Justice Oil

Solomon's seal root

Master root

Licorice root

Victory over an Enemy

Call on God and Moses, and pray Exodus 15 V 1-19 over a white candle. Do this work for five days.

> *1 Then sang Moses and the children of Israel this song unto the LORD, and spake, saying, I will sing unto the LORD, for he hath triumphed gloriously: the horse and his rider hath he thrown into the sea.*
>
> *2 The LORD is my strength and song, and he is become my salvation: he is my God, and I will prepare him an habitation; my father's God, and I will exalt him.*
>
> *3 The LORD is a man of war; the LORD is his name.*
>
> *4 Pharaoh's chariots and his host hath he cast into the sea: his chosen captains also are drowned in the Red sea.*
>
> *5 The depths have covered them: they sank into the bottom as a stone.*
>
> *6 Thy right hand, O LORD, is become glorious in power: thy right hand, O LORD, hath dashed in pieces the enemy.*
>
> *7 And in the greatness of thine excellency thou hast overthrown them that rose up against thee: thou sentest forth thy wrath, which consumed them as stubble.*
>
> *8 And with the blast of thy nostrils the waters were gathered together, the floods stood upright*

as an heap, and the depths were congealed in the heart of the sea.

9 The enemy said, I will pursue, I will overtake, I will divide the spoil; my lust shall be satisfied upon them; I will draw my sword, my hand shall destroy them.

10 Thou didst blow with thy wind, the sea covered them: they sank as lead in the mighty waters.

11 Who is like unto thee, O LORD, among the gods? Who is like thee, glorious in holiness, fearful in praises, doing wonders?

12 Thou stretchedst out thy right hand, the earth swallowed them.

13 Thou in thy mercy hast led forth the people which thou hast redeemed: thou hast guided them in thy strength unto thy holy habitation.

14 The people shall hear, and be afraid: sorrow shall take hold on the inhabitants of Palestina.

15 Then the dukes of Edom shall be amazed; the mighty men of Moab, trembling shall take hold upon them; all the inhabitants of Canaan shall melt away.

16 Fear and dread shall fall upon them; by the greatness of thine arm they shall be as still as a stone; till thy people pass over, O LORD, till the people pass over, which thou hast purchased.

17 Thou shalt bring them in, and plant them in the mountain of thine inheritance, in the place, O LORD, which thou hast made for thee to dwell in, in the Sanctuary, O LORD, which thy hands have established.

18 The LORD shall reign forever and ever.

19 For the horse of Pharaoh went in with his chariots and with his horsemen into the sea, and the LORD brought again the waters of the sea upon them; but the children of Israel went on dry land in the midst of the sea.

Victory

Moses will come to our aid when we call on him against our enemies. Dress a purple candle with olive oil, light the candle, and call on Moses and petition him to give you victory over your enemies. Pray Numbers 10 V 9 and 35 over the candle three times. Do this daily until the candle burns out. It needs to be done for at least seven days.

9 And if ye go to war in your land against the enemy that oppresseth you; then ye shall blow an alarm with the trumpets; and ye shall be remembered before the LORD your God, and ye shall be saved from your enemies.

35 And it came to pass, when the ark set forward, that Moses said, Rise up, LORD, and let thine enemies be scattered; and let them hate thee flee before thee.

Justice Work

In Judges 16, we see that Delia found Samson's secret and he was taken prisoner. They put his eyes out. In Judges 16 V 27-30 Samson screams for justice because they took his sight. This is a very hard work; it should not be done just because you feel someone has slighted you. You should only do this work if you have good reason. The setup to use with this work is the cross. Alternate your vigils two red and two purple for the cross. For the center use a black vigil.

I personally don't place a name in the wax of this central vigil. I write "those who have wronged me." This way you don't hit the wrong person. Dress the black vigil with olive oil. Hold the vigil up high out in front of you; call on God and in a strong voice ask that justice be served. Light your cross setup and on each one say "justice WILL be served." Light your black vigil and pray Judges 16 V 27-30 over the setup three times. Repeat this daily until all the vigils have burned out.

> *27 Now the house was full of men and women; and all the lords of the Philistines were there; and there were upon the roof about three thousand men and women, that beheld while Samson made sport.*
>
> *28 And Samson called unto the LORD, and said, O LORD God, remember me, I pray thee, and strengthen me, I pray thee, only this once, O GOD, that I may be at once avenged of the Philistines for my two eyes.*

*29 And Samson took hold of the two middle pil-
lars upon which the house stood, and on which it
was borne up, of the one with his right hand, and
of the other with his left.*

*30 And Samson said, Let me die with the Philis-
tines. And he bowed himself with all his might;
and the house fell upon the lords, and upon all
the people that were therein. So the dead which he
slew at his death were more than they which he
slew in his life.*

Recipes for Removing

Removing Oil

Lemon balm

Lemon essential oil

Master of the Woods

Hotfoot

There are times when we have to be heavy-handed. Some folks just
don't get the message that we want to be left alone, or they can't
mind their own business and seem to thrive off of making others
miserable. When this happens, it is time to send them stepping. If
you find yourself in this situation get a small baby food jar; tear out
Genesis 31 V 13 from the Bible and write the person's name on it four
times going away from you. Place it in the jar.

Pray Genesis 31 V 13 into the jar before you close it. Call the person's name after you pray the verse. Do this three times before you close the jar. Once you have the jar closed, shake it as hard as you can while you pray Genesis 31 V 13. At the end of the verse say the person's name. Light a tealight on top of the jar and let it burn out. Pray your petition over the tealight. Follow these instructions daily for twenty-one days. On the twenty-second day throw the jar in running water.

> *13 I am the God of Bethel, where thou anointedst the pillar, and where thou vowedst a vow unto me: now arise, get thee out from this land, and return unto the land of thy kindred.*

Blockbuster Work

There are times when it seems our way has been blocked and we are bound down and can't move forward. In Exodus 3 V 18-20 we see that Moses can stretch out his hand by the power of God and set you free. Moses will remove what is holding you down. Get an orange seven-day candle, and wipe yourself off with the candle from head to toe. Then hold the candle up to your mouth, and call on God and Moses. Ask Moses to set you free from the bonds that are holding you down. Pray Exodus 3 V 18-20 over the candle three times, then light the candle. Go daily three times a day and say your prayer over the candle; each time petitioning Moses to set you free. Do this until the candle has burned out.

> *18 And they shall hearken to thy voice: and thou shalt come, thou and the elders of Israel, unto the king of Egypt, and ye shall say unto him, The*

LORD God of the Hebrews hath met with us: and now let us go, we beseech thee, three days' journey into the wilderness, that we may sacrifice to the LORD our God.

19 And I am sure that the king of Egypt will not let you go, no, not by a mighty hand.

20 And I will stretch out my hand, and smite Egypt with all my wonders which I will do in the midst thereof: and after that he will let you go.

Hotfoot Work

Hotfoot should never be taken lightly. This work should be done when all else fails. If you find yourself in a situation where hotfoot is needed, then this powerful work is for you. In Numbers 33 V 40-48 we see that when the children of Israel headed for Canaan, King Arad ran. He went from place to place, so these verses are good for hotfoot work. Make a hotfoot jar and pray these verses over the jar. After each verse call the target's name and tell them where you want them to end up. Burn a tealight on the jar daily. Do this work for twenty-one days, then throw the jar in running water.

40 And king Arad the Canaanite, which dwelt in the south in the land of Canaan, heard of the coming of the children of Israel.

41 And they departed from mount Hor, and pitched in Zalmonah.

42 And they departed from Zalmonah, and pitched in Punon.

43 And they departed from Punon, and pitched in Oboth.

44 And they departed from Oboth, and pitched in Ijeabarim, in the border of Moab.

45 And they departed from Iim, and pitched in Dibongad.

46 And they removed from Dibongad, and encamped in Almondiblathaim.

47 And they removed from Almondiblataim, and pitched in the mountains of Abarim, before Nebo.

48 And they departed from the mountains of Abarim, and pitched in the plains of Moab by Jordan near Jericho.

Recipes for Success

Crown of Success Oil

Bergamot

Deer's-tongue

High John

Master of the Woods

Solomon's seal root

Crown of Success

In Joshua 1 V 5–9 God promises us success and prosperity. Take these verses out of the Bible, and burn them to ash. Mix the ash with a pinch of coriander seed. Write your name in the wax of an orange vigil, then load the mixture into the candle. Call on God. Hold the candle up to your mouth, and pray these verses into the candle. Light the candle, and continue to pray these verses to it until the candle burns out.

> *5 There shall not any man be able to stand before thee all the days of thy life: as I was with Moses, so I will be with thee: I will not fail thee, nor for-sake thee.*
>
> *6 Be strong and of a good courage: for unto this people shalt thou divide for an inheritance the land, which I sware unto their fathers to give them.*
>
> *7 Only be thou strong and very courageous, that thou mayest observe to do according to all the law, which Moses my servant commanded thee: turn not from it to the right hand or to the left, that thou mayest prosper withersoever thou goest.*
>
> *8 This book of the law shall not depart out of thy mouth; but thou shalt meditate therein day and night, that thou mayest observe to do according to all that is written therein: for then thou shalt make thy way prosperous, and then thou shalt have good success.*
>
> *9 Have not I commanded thee? Be strong and of a good courage; be not afraid, neither be thou dis-mayed: for the LORD thy God is with thee whith-ersoever thou goest.*

I hope these recipes serve you well and give you an idea of how to make your own oils.

Washes and Powders

Washes

I wanted to share a few washes and powder recipes with y'all. Not many folks nowadays make real old-school washes. Most of what you can get is not much more than colored water. It is easy to make your own floor washes and sprays. They don't have a long shelf life, but you can make small batches as needed.

All you have to do is add your roots and herbs to a pot of boiling water. Let them boil for a few minutes, then turn the fire off and cover them. Leave them to steep until they cool, then you can strain them. Your wash or spray is ready. Remember to pray over them while they are steeping. After you strain the wash, you can sprinkle the roots and herbs you used around your door stoop.

Money Drawing Wash

Shredded money

Cinnamon

Blue flag

Peaceful Home Wash

Bloodroot

Bay leaf

Pinch of salt

Rule the Roost Wash

Licorice

Calamus

Master of the Woods

Blessing Wash

Rosemary

Sandalwood

Marjoram

Better Business Wash

Solomon's seal root

Thyme

High John the Conqueror root

Money Magnet Wash

Shredded money

A large magnet

Gumbo filé

Attraction Wash

Large magnet

Sassafras

Lovage

Destroy a Crossed Condition

> Frankincense
>
> Myrrh
>
> Angelica root

Conjure Powders

Powders today are nothing more than a base powder like talc or cornstarch that powdered herbs are added into if they have herbs in them at all. In the old days powders were made from dirts and pounded herbs and roots, but in the world of commercial Hoodoo it's hard to find old-school products like these. When you gather your dirts, make sure you pay for them—drop a few coins in the hole where you got it. Just like you don't work for free, neither does Spirit. The key is to know which herbs do what, where to gather the dirt, and to remember that prayer is very important if you want your powders to be a success. You can powder your own herbs with a small covered grinder. Here are a few recipes.

Money Drawing Powder

> Sassafras
>
> Money burned to ash
>
> Magnetic sand

Money Drawing Powder 2

> Money burned to ash
>
> Cinnamon
>
> Magnetic sand

Money Drawing Powder 3

Shredded money burned to ash

Salt

Bay leaves

Love Powder

Adam-and-eve root

Damiana

Sugar

Love Powder 2

Catnip

Rose

Dirt dauber nest

Love Powder 3

Crossroads dirt

Lovage root

Lavender

Dominating Powder

Licorice

Calamus

Dirt dauber nest

Peaceful Home

Lavender

Basil

Bay leaf

Protection Powder

Dirt from a church

Rue

Chamomile

CONJURING
HOUSEHOLD PLANTS

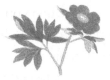

Lots of folks know about working with roots and herbs, but working with houseplants and trees is dying out as elders pass and the information is lost. Conjure work is not just roots, herbs, and spells. It is also about maintaining the home and the community, and plants play a big part in the old ways of working. I did not want to do an herbal without adding houseplants and how to work with them to bring prosperity, health, luck, and protection into the home. And there are also some plants that can cause crossed conditions and stop gossip. A lot of this knowledge is not being shared. I learned to do the work through stories and hands-on training from my elders, so a lot of what I share can be told in stories that help us remember the work.

When I was growing up, yards were swept every Saturday, and no work was done on Sunday. My grandma, mama, and aunties made the brooms we used to sweep the yard. Back in that time not a lot of yards had grass in them; they were mostly dirt. I learned to sweep the yard when I was young. You may be thinking: What is so hard about sweeping a yard? Well, trust me, it was not that easy for me at first. This lesson also taught me how to sweep inside the house. My grandma was very strict on how she wanted the yard swept: You had to sweep with one sweep, then pick up the broom and do another sweep. There was no sweeping back and forth. When I was young, I didn't understand why you had to sweep like that, but I do now. When you sweep back and forth, all you are doing is stirring up any mess that has been laid, but when you sweep in a full sweep, you are moving it in one direction away from you.

The reason folks swept their yards was to keep them clean but also to make sure no tricks were laid for them to get into. They washed the stoops for the same reason. Because there was dirt in the yard, it would have been easy for someone to drop a trick in the yard or on the stoop and you would never be the wiser because you would have thought it was just dirt.

Growing up, I wasn't given a reason why we had to sweep the yard on Saturday or why the stoops were washed every morning; it was just something we did when we were at grandma's house. When we were home, my mama tended to all that.

I can still close my eyes and see my grandma's house. It sat back from the dirt road, and she had a line of pine trees between her house and the road. Pine trees are good for protection and cleansing. On each side of the front door stoop she had large pots full of touch-me-nots, or what some call jewelweed. I loved those plants, and I got in a lot of trouble for messing with them. The touch-me-not is a very powerful plant to have in the front of the house or around a doorway. The name gives you the plant's power, but it isn't just about the name. When you touch the little seedpods that grow on the plant, they burst open and the seeds go flying. That's why

I stayed in trouble with my grandma: I loved busting those seeds. Touch-me-nots are not only good for protection, but they also have healing properties. Many old-timey plants are given names that will let you know how to work with them.

The reason the touch-me-not is good for protection is because of those bursting seeds: they burst open with some force away from the plant. So, if someone is throwing at you, the plant will keep the energy at bay just like the hull of the seed protects the seed. A lot of plants do different types of work: some protect, some heal, some do both like the touch-me-not. This plant is good for bugbites, poison ivy, and other rashes that itch. You can break off a small piece of the plant and then you milk the healing juice out of the stem and put it right on the bite or rash. It will help stop the itching. You can also make a tincture or even a salve that will help.

I am gonna share my recipes for both with you. For this tincture I like to use witch hazel. Witch hazel has its own healing properties. When I was a teenager, my mama made us clean our faces with witch hazel, and I never had an issue with my face breaking out. Your skin feels refreshed.

Bugbite Tincture, Salve, or Oil

To make the tincture, you will need a good-size bunch of touch-me-not stems, since the stems hold the healing milk. You need a quart mason jar with a lid and enough witch hazel to cover the touch-me-nots. Make sure that your work area is clean and the jar has been cleaned well. Gather your greens and wash them well. I have a copper bowl I place plants I am working with in. Put the plants in a bowl—please do not use plastic. Place a white stick candle in the center of the plants, light it, and pray the Isaiah 38 V 16 over the plant at least three times before the candle burns out. Say the prayer and then your petition.

> *O Lord, by these things men live, and in all these things is the life of my spirit: so, wilt thou recover me, and make me to live.*

When the candle burns out, then bend the stems and plant matter and place them in the jar. Once you have them in the jar, pour the witch hazel in the jar, making sure it covers the plant. Blow three breaths into the jar, and say the prayer and your petition into the jar. Then place the lid on the jar. Put the tincture in a cool dark place. Every three days take the jar out and burn a white stick candle on top of the jar. Say your prayer and petition over the jar three times before the candle burns out. Then place the jar back where you had it. This should be done for the first twenty-one days. Once the twenty-one days are up, you need to leave the tincture put away for at least another three weeks. Then it should be ready.

Once it is ready, you need to strain all the plant matter out of the tincture. I use a strainer on the first strain, and then I use a white handkerchief on the second strain. Some folks like to use cheese-cloth, but I have found that plant matter can still get through the cheesecloth. So for me a handkerchief works better. You can use whatever you have on hand as long as you get all the plant mat-ter out of the tincture so it doesn't cause mold and ruin it. You can either leave it in the mason jar or place it in a small spray bottle and apply as needed. It should have a long shelf life. As with everything, use caution and make sure you are not allergic to the plant or the witch hazel.

You can also make a salve or an oil if you don't like the smell of the tincture. To make the salve you will need some olive oil, beeswax, vitamin E oil, some containers to hold the salve, and some type of essential oil. I like to use lavender oil because it relaxes and soothes. You need a large clean mason jar and a pot that you can use as a double boiler. Wash the plant really well, making sure there are no bugs or dirt left on the plant. Once the plant is cleaned, place it in a bowl with a white stick candle. Light the candle and pray Jeremiah 33 V 6 over the plant along with your petition. Say the prayer and petition three times over the plant while the candle is burning.

> *Behold, I will bring it health and cure, and I will*
> *cure them, and will reveal unto them the abun-*
> *dance of peace and truth.*

Once the candle burns out and the prayers are done, add the plant to the jar, and cover the ingredients with the olive oil. Now it is time to place the jar in the double boiler.

Fill the pot half full of water and place it on the stove on a high heat. Let the water come to a hard boil, then lower the flame and place the mason jar in the water with the lid off. The oil needs to cook for about six hours on a low heat. Once the oil is done, remove the jar from the double boiler and strain the oil well the same way you did for the tincture. I pour mine back into the jar until I have the rest of the ingredients ready to mix together. I wrap the jar with a hand towel to keep the oil warm while I heat up the rest of my ingredients.

I have made salves for so long I don't measure anything anymore. I just eye it and add it to the mix. Place the beeswax in a small jar and put it in the double boiler to melt; it should do that pretty fast. Don't overheat the wax or it will break down. You can also melt a little coco butter or shea butter with the beeswax and add it to the salve. Once the ingredients are melted, combine this with your olive oil and put it back in the double boiler, stirring it lightly to mix it all together. You can add whatever essential oil you chose at this time. Make sure it is mixed well or the oil will sit on top of the salve. Once it is mixed well, remove it from the heat and pour it into your containers.

Once the salve sets, you can put the lids on it. If you put the lids on before it is set, moisture will form on top of the salve. When the salve is ready, place the containers in a cross setup of four white stick candles. The setup should be top to bottom and left to right to nail down the healing of the salve. Say the prayer and petition over the candles as they burn. Once the candles go out, the salve is ready to use.

Side Note

Some folks don't like what I call a flat salve; they prefer a kind of whipped cream. If you would rather have the whipped cream effect, then you will need to pour all the ingredients in a bowl and use a whisk to whip the ingredients just like you are whisking an egg white. When it is fluffy enough, you can spoon it into your container. This method will take more containers than just pouring out a flat salve. Also remember if you get your fire too high trying to rush the process, it will break down the ingredients. This type of work takes time and patience.

If you do not want to make the tincture or salve for whatever reason, you can also make an oil that will do the same thing. When I was coming up, olive oil was the oil that was worked with. It is a healing oil within itself, but back in the day, that is what my elders taught me to work with. Spiritual oils were cooked in a double boiler on a very low heat depending on the ingredients. It could take days to make an oil, then it had to be worked before it could be used. Nowadays everyone is too busy, and they want everything to be fast and easy. This is one of the reasons the old ways are dying out: nobody makes time anymore to learn the right way of doing things. To make the oil, you follow the same instructions as the tincture and the salve with the plant and oil in the double boiler. Once the oil has simmered for about six hours, you can strain the plant material out of it. Then you can add your essential oil and vitamin E oil to the jar. Stir it in well, and add it back to the double boiler for twenty minutes or so, slightly stirring it every so often to make sure all the ingredients are mixed well. Then you can either leave it in the jar or place it in small bottles. Then you place the containers in a cross setup of four white stick candles. The setup should be top to bottom and left to right to nail down the healing of the oil. Say the prayer and petition over the candles as they burn. Once the candles go out, the oil is ready to use.

The old ways of doing the work take longer, but the results are so much more powerful. Here is something to think about: Do you realize that every time you do an old work all the ancestors who did that work come when you are fixing the ingredients? You are following in their footsteps. Sometimes the old ways are the better ways!

Working Houseplants

This list is most definitely not a complete reckoning of houseplants that can be worked with for Conjure, but this is my list of plants that I have or still do work with.

Plants are a powerful way to work for a few reasons. First, they are a living thing, so as long as you keep the plant alive, the work will live. If you let the plant die, the work dies. Also, the stronger the roots get, the stronger the work becomes and the stronger the hold on the target will become as the roots grow around the work. I wrote a little about this in *Hoodoo Your Love*. This is one of the first types of work I learned to do. The old folks say, "Plant the seed, the tree will grow." The same is true about planting a work.

Plants are also a barrier between our world and the spiritual world; I say this because if someone is trying to cross you up or sends a spirit after you, most of the time it is gonna hit the plants first. You have to remember that spirit can't tell the difference between a person or a plant because we are both living beings! This is why in the old days you would see a lot of flower gardens in patches on either side of the house; you would also see old farming tools thrown in the yards or leaning against the house or a tree. It wasn't because the folks were lazy and didn't clean up: it is because old tools were made out of iron and iron protects! Folks would leave old tractors that no longer worked in the front of their fields. Again, this wasn't laziness; it was protection. Nowadays they will call the county on you if you try to do this. Folks cannot seem to mind their own business in today's world!

Rules for Planting

There are just a few rules when planting. I was never taught to work by the moon except when it came to cutting my hair and planting. If you plant a plant when the moon is going down or when the sun is setting, that plant will struggle to grow. This would be the time to plant when you are trying to stop or remove a target. When the moon is growing and before the sun sits high in the sky at noon are the time to plant to bring something to you. This works with all plants—herbs, roots, and household plants. I cannot stress enough that if you are doing love, peaceful home, money works, or any type of positive work, if the plant dies so will the work! So like any other type of conjure work you have to actually do the work: you can't just plant the plant or seeds and leave it on its own. You have to work the plant.

I will reuse old pots and potting soil to plant my regular plants, but if I am conjuring a plant, I usually buy a new pot and fresh potting soil. I've written a little about this before and have taught some of my longtime hands-on students how to work with plants, but this is the first time I have ever really given step-by-step details in a book. I feel that it is time to write this down lest it be lost. My family holds this knowledge, but they will never share it outside of the family. They do works, but it is for them. They don't conjure for other folks.

When I decide to plant a new plant for conjure work, there are always things that I do. If I am doing the work to pull something to me, once I have my potting soil ready to take the plant that I am going to transplant, I take the plant out of the pot. I hold the roots in my hands and blow three breaths onto the roots. Then I spit on the roots. Our breath and our spit hold our spirit, so this links you and the plant together. At this time also say my prayer and my petition over the roots. Then I will set the plant aside and get the pot ready to add the plant to it. It all depends on what type of work I am doing as to what I add to the pot.

Fixing a Plant for Prosperity

For example, I can tell you about the work that I did to keep prosperity coming into the home. When I did this work, I painted the container that the work and plant would go into myself. I used an empty coffee container, and I painted a face on it. I took a photo of my front door, printed it out, and placed it in the bottom of the container. On top of the photo I put a two-dollar bill, and on top of the bill I placed a magnet. You have to remember that like begets like, so if you want to draw money into your home doing any type of conjure work, you need to work with real money. The reason I took a photo of my front door and added it and put the money on top of it is so that the money will flow in the door. The magnet on top of the money was also to pull the money in the door. Once I had the personal items in the bottom of the planter, I put a little bit of the potting soil on top of it—probably about an inch deep.

I said my prayer and petition over the soil in the pot, and I once again blew three breaths over the soil and spit on the soil. After that the soil and the pot were ready for the plant. I once again held the plant by the roots and the soil that was holding the roots together and said my prayer and my petition again. Then I added the plant to the pot and covered the roots with the remaining fixed soil. I held the leaves of the plant in both of my hands and said my prayer and petition again over them. Then I gave the leaves three more breaths. Lastly, I gave the plant a good drink of water. I sat there for a while just talking to the plant and giving thanks for the work that it will be doing for me. I talk to that plant every day and I say my prayer and my petition over it daily.

These are the basics of how to fix a plant to draw something to you. Dirts from the four corners of your yard and the front and back door give spirits a map to the work. The life of the plant pulls Spirit in, and as the plant grows, the power within the plant will grow so the work becomes stronger as time goes on. I always get the dirt from the four corners of my yard and from the front and back door stoops for all positive works.

Fixing a Plant for Shut Your Mouth

If I am doing a darker work such as shut your mouth or a souring work on someone, the work is a little different. You would not want to put your personal items in this type of work, so you wouldn't add anything that concerns you. That means you don't breathe or spit on it. And you don't gather dirt from your property. You only add things that have to do with the target. For example, I'll give you a shut your mouth work that I put on targets some years ago. When you do a shut your mouth, traditionally you add red pepper to the work and usually something bitter to sour their mouth. You can also do this type of work with a plant. You need a plant that is hot like a jalapeño bush.

When I did this work, I bought a small jalapeño plant so as the plant grew and became hotter, the work would grow and become hotter. For this type of work I use the nastiest planter that I have on hand. I will print up a photo of the target, and add any personal items of theirs that I have in the bottom of container. Normally when you transplant a new plant, you move it from one container to the next as it grows bigger, so the plant doesn't struggle to grow to fit the container; but for this type of work you want the plant to have a little struggle because it makes the target have struggles. Now this work will not only heat up the target, but it's also going to sour their mouth. You need a lemon, a photo of the target, some red pepper, and four needles. Cut the lemon into four pieces longways. Place the target's photo in the lemon and cover all the pieces of lemon with the red pepper. Then you put the lemon back together like a puzzle with the photo and the red pepper on the inside. Use the needles to hold the lemon pieces in place. While you are pinning the lemon back together, say your petition over the lemon.

I usually say something like every time you speak my name or have ill will against me, your mouth will burn and your day will turn sour. But you can say whatever petition fits your situation. Sometimes in the past I have added dirt from other places to this work. It all depends on the reason I am doing the work. Just remember that you and only you are responsible for every work that you do. All works of this type should be justified. If you are unjustly throwing at a target, the work can and will come back on you. I'm pretty sure you don't want to get hit with your own work. So just be sure that the work fits the situation that you are dealing with.

Add some of the potting soil to your container to cover the bottom of the container. Then place the lemon inside the potting soil so that the lemon is upside down; this will also cause confusion to the target. Add another layer of potting soil and cover the lemon completely. Then take your pepper plant and hold the roots in your hand. Be sure not to let your breath get on those roots as you say your prayer and petition over the roots three times. Now add the plant to the potting soil and finish covering the roots with the remaining soil. Name the plant after the target. Give the plant a good drink of water, and then call the target's name and tell the target what is going to happen. Talk to that plant daily and make sure that you water the plant. Remember, jalapeño plants need to be watered at least twice a week.

Being Justified

Before we move on to the plants and how to work with certain plants, I want to make sure that you understand that this work is not all love and light. The ancestors did not have the luxury of love and light; they lived in a bitter, harsh world where just looking at a white person in the face could get you killed. I know that folks nowadays try to forget about slavery and where this work comes from. If you are going to take on the responsibility of doing this work, then you really need to understand that this work comes on the back of those who were treated like less than animals. I know that some folks get upset about my writing about this sometimes, but I'm here to share valuable information that is being lost and not to hold hands and sugarcoat anything. This work comes from blood, bones, death, and suffering—so yes, some of these works that you will find in this section might be what some consider harsh. If you feel like parts of this work are too harsh and not for you, then don't do it. But if you feel like any of the hard work is necessary in your world, then just know that you and you alone are responsible for your own actions. Just because you know how to do something doesn't mean you have to do it: it's all your choice. I am what they call a two-headed conjure worker because I do the types of work that I feel are justified and that Spirit gives me permission to do.

You should never do any type of work no matter what kind it is without doing some type of divination first. Sometimes Spirit doesn't want us to step in and do work. If you do divination on a job and Spirit tells you not to do the work, then don't do it. If you decide to do the work anyway, then that is on you. Remember, everything costs something; nothing is free in this life.

Dedicating a Plant

There are times when you may want to dedicate a plant to a certain thing or spirit. If you decide to do this, you need to make sure that you take special care of that plant. For example, I have a money tree that I dedicated to St. Peter. St. Peter holds the keys to the gates and unlocks all doors. The plant sits next to St. Peter's house that sits behind the work in my living room. We have to remember that plants are living things, so they need to be watered and fed in order for them to keep living. When you dedicate a plant to a spirit, you are making a contract to that spirit that you will do the best you can do by that plant and take care of it and in return the spirit will bless you with whatever you fix the plant for. When I dedicate a plant to a certain spirit, I will always buy a fresh plant. I won't use cuttings from other plants. And I also buy a fresh container for that plant. If you decide that you would like to dedicate a plant for St. Peter, follow the instructions here.

You don't necessarily have to have a money plant. You can have a cactus for protection, maybe an aloe for healing, or even a sweet potato to draw in prosperity. It all depends on you and what you are trying to do. St. Peter helps with many different things. He can open the doors or close them. He can heal. He can draw in prosperity and much more. It just all depends on what you are petitioning him for. For this example, I am going to share with you how to fix a cactus for protection of your home by dedicating it to St. Peter. When you pot a cactus, it uses a different type of soil. You will need potting soil, sand, and some small pebbles. You need to add the pebbles into the mix so that the roots of the cactus don't rot in case you overwater the plant. Cacti are easy to take care of, so if you don't have a green thumb and you want to dedicate a plant, this would be a good one.

It is important to remember that we assume nothing when we are dealing with Spirit. Before you dedicate a plant to a spirit, you need to first do a divination with either a pendulum, cards, or whatever tool you usually work with and ask that spirit if they will work through that plant for you for whatever condition you are petitioning for. If you get no for an answer, then it could be they don't want to work with you in that situation, or it could be you picked the wrong plant. So, if you get a no on one plant, ask Spirit to show you the best plant for the work you are petitioning them for. This is where your gift of discernment is really needed. If you go against Spirit and give them the plant that you want to give them, it is a possibility that the plant will die or the work will not come to fruition. It is very important with any type of conjure work for which you jump in with both feet that you do divination first. Remember that not everything is meant for you. Just because something worked for someone else does not mean that that exact same thing will work for you. Divination and discernment are the key to success in this work. Spirit always holds the key to our success. Spirit holds the power for failure or success in all we do. You need to always remember to ask Spirit before you move forward; it makes life a lot easier.

When you are ready to do your planting, you will need dirt from the four corners of the property you live on and dirt from the front and the back door. This dirt will be mixed in the potting soil and the sand. Mix the dirts together well and add a few of the pebbles in the dirt mixture. Take a photo of your front door and a photo of your family if you want to, and place them on top of a thin layer of the dirt mixture inside the pot. Then put another thin layer of the dirt mixture in the pot so the photos are completely covered. Now place a small thin layer of pebbles on top of the dirt mixture. Blow three breaths over the mixture and petition St. Peter to protect your family and your home against all those who would try to harm you.

Take the cactus out of the container and place it on top of the small pebbles. Fill the pot up with the rest of the dirt mixture. You can either place the plant in a sunny window by the front door or on the door stoop at the front door.

The Houseplants, A to Z

I don't know the correct name for all the plants that I have or have worked with over the years. I only know what they are called in the world I live in. I'm sure that if you do some research, you can find their scientific names, but I am going to use the names that I know them by. Sometimes the names will give you an idea of what the plant can be worked with for. For example, mother-in-law's tongue can be worked to stop gossip, to shut someone's mouth, and to keep folks out of your business. The milky substance that comes from the plant when a piece is broke off is bitter, so therefore, it would leave a bitter taste in the target's mouth. Another plant would be the touch-me-nots—just the name explains that all. Or what about the weeping willow? You immediately get the idea that the tree is crying. So the weeping willow would be a good tree to work with to either stop someone from crying or make someone cry—it all depends on the prayer and the petition and the work that is done. One last example is an iron plant. We all know that iron is powerful. You cannot break iron. The only way to destroy iron is with fire. So an iron plant could be worked with for protection, low self-esteem, or finances. Many plants do many different kinds of work; they all have different characteristics and different personalities. It really all depends on the need and the prayer and petition. With that being said, let's move on to the plants.

Aloe

The aloe vera plant is well-known for its healing properties, but this plant can also be worked with for prosperity, protection, and to hide you from an enemy. You may be thinking: how does this plant hide me from an enemy? It's all in the gel inside the plant. In order for an enemy to get to you, they would have to get through the thick gel that makes up the aloe. If you needed to hide yourself from an enemy, you would need two pieces of the plant, a photo of yourself or your home, and some red cotton thread. Place the photo in between the two pieces of aloe vera. Then take the red thread and wrap the two pieces of plant while stating your prayer and your petition that the plant hide you from all your enemies. You can then take that packet and either put it away in a safe place or place it in a pot and plant a new aloe vera on top of it. Then you place the plant inside your home where it can get enough sunlight to continue to grow. Speak to the plant daily and take very good care of this plant as it is working for you.

You can also work with an aloe vera plant to draw in prosperity. If you are going to pull prosperity into the whole household, then you need to take a photo of the front door of the home. Gather dirt from the four corners of the property and dirt from each side of the front door stoop; then you mix this dirt with a good potting soil. Put a thin layer of potting soil in the bottom of the pot, then you place the photo facing upward. Make sure that the photo is put in the right way because if you place the photo in that pot facedown, you are going to block the whole household's prosperity. Cover the photo with a thin layer of dirt and then hold the roots of the plant in your hands and say your prayer and petition. Give the plant a good spit. Take three quarters and stick them in the roots of the plant; be gentle because you do not want to bruise the roots. Place the roots in the pot and cover them the rest of the way with your potting soil. Give the plant a cool drink of water and say your prayer and petition over the plant. Be sure to give the plant thanks for its help. Also make sure that you spend time with the plant at least once a week. As the plant grows, your prosperity should grow.

Angel Plant

The angel plant can be worked with for protection and guidance. You could dedicate this plant to archangel Michael for protection. You would need to do a divination to make sure that St. Michael would accept the work. St. Michael is a warrior. You have to remember that angels are not these sugary fluffy beings at our command. They are powerful warriors and should be shown respect. If you would like to petition St. Michael for this work, then do the right thing and ask permission. Once you get the okay through your divination, you take your photo after you have done a spiritual bath or a brush-off with a candle and burned that candle. This is called a clean photo. Place the photo of you between two novena cards that have St. Michael depicted on them. Use a red cotton thread to bind the novena cards together. You will then need four red stick candles. Say your petition over each of the candles and then place them in a cross setup going top to bottom, left to right. Place your packet in the center of this, and petition St. Michael to protect you and to guide you. Light the candles in the same order that you set them down, and as you light each candle repeat your prayer and your petition.

While the candles burn, you will need to get a red flowerpot, soil, and your plant. Place about two inches of dirt in the pot. Then after the candles burn out, place the prayer cards on top of the dirt along with the leftover wax from the candles. Cover those items up with another layer of soil. Now it's time to add your plant. Hold the roots in your hands and say your prayer and your petition over them. You should do this at least three times. Then place the plant in the soil and cover up the roots. Make sure to water the plant well and give thanks to St. Michael for his protection. If you have a St. Michael altar set up, you can place your plant on his altar. If you don't have an altar, then you can set the plant in a low-lying area. Make sure that you don't overwater the plant or that it doesn't get too much sunlight. Too much sunlight will burn the plant. Make sure that you take very good care of this plant and that you speak with St. Michael at least twice a week to give your thanks. There are many works that could be done with this plant. This is just an example to get you started.

Angel's-Trumpet

First, let me make it very clear that the angel's-trumpet is a very poisonous plant and should *never* be eaten. The whole plant is poisonous! Still, these are beautiful plants, and they grow fast. They need to be planted in soil that has good drainage, and they do well in pots. These plants grow flowers on them that are shaped like trumpets. If you believe in the book of Revelation, then you know that an angel will blow the trumpet on Judgment Day. In Revelation 8 we see that there will be seven trumpets blown and the last one is the call to judgment. That's when folks pay for the things that they've done wrong in this life.

Keeping that in mind, there is a work that can be done with the angel's-trumpet plant to bring justice against an enemy for the wrong they may have done you. This work will bring forth the judgment of their peers and bring to light their wrongdoing. It is like you will find in Revelation 11 V 15-18.

> *15 Then the seventh angel sounded: And there were loud voices in heaven, saying, "The kingdoms of this world have become the kingdoms of our Lord and of His Christ, and He shall reign forever and ever!"*

> *16 And the twenty-four elders who sat before God on their thrones fell on their faces and worshiped God,*

> *17 Saying: "We give You thanks, O Lord God Almighty, the One who is and who was and who is to come, because You have taken Your great power and reigned.*

> *18 The nations were angry, and Your wrath has come, and the time of the dead, that they should be judged, and that You should reward Your servants the prophets and the saints, and those who fear Your name, small and great, and should destroy those who destroy the earth."*

I was taught to tear a chapter and verse directly out of the Bible to be worked with. I know that some folks have a fear of doing this even if they are Christians. The thing that I learned as a young conjure woman is that you cannot destroy the words of the Bible. Even if you set them on fire, you will still be able to read the words in that ash; they cannot be destroyed. So with that being said, you can either tear out Revelation 11 V 15-18 or you can print it out. Take Revelation 11 V 15-18, and write the target's name on it three times.

Three is a very powerful number. It is written over and over how things in Revelation come in threes—and really throughout the whole Bible. Once you have the name written down three times, write your petition over the name. You simply need to write a short statement using the power words of what you are seeking from this work: justice and that the target's actions be revealed.

You will need an angel's-trumpet plant, potting soil, dirt from a courthouse where justice is served, and your petition. Put a little bit of potting soil in a pot and then lay your petition on top of it. Burn a tealight on top of the petition while praying Revelation 11 V 15-18 over the petition three times. Let the tealight burn out. Once the light goes out, remove the tealight's metal container from the planter. Cover the petition with the dirt from the courthouse and a little bit of potting soil. Hold the roots of the angel's-trumpet plant in both hands, and pray the Revelation verses over them and speak your petition three times. Then cover the roots with potting soil. Every day for twenty-one days go and say the prayer and your petition over the plant three times a day. At the end of the twenty-one days go say your prayer and petition over the plant every three days. You will repeat the prayer and petition three times each time you go and say the prayers. You will do this until justice has been served.

Cactus

Everyone knows that the cactus is very protective due to the thorns. The thorns poke and draw blood, so therefore it is a good plant to have in the front of your house. When we first moved into our house thirty-some years ago, I had a large cactus garden on the left-hand side of my house and a large rosebush on the right side of the house.

The first bad hurricane that we had destroyed my cactus bed, but my rosebush is still standing.

Cacti are known for pulling water out of the ground. This is one way they survive in the desert. Even one cactus is better than none for protection. They are also very low-maintenance plants. If you don't have a lot of time or you are not good with growing plants, then the cactus might be a good plant for you to grow and to work with. The thorns that grow on the larger cactus can be worked with to nail an enemy down or to cross an enemy up.

If you have an enemy that just will not leave you alone, you can get two thorns off of a large cactus and the enemy's photo. You run the thorns through the head of the photo with the photo being placed upside down. Place one thorn going downward and the other one crossing. When you place each of the thorns into the photo, say your prayer and your petition. Once this is done, place the photo in a candle setup with the head of the target upside down and petition the spirit of the plant to hold your enemy down. Once the candles burn out, take the photo and nail it up against the wall with the head facing downward. There are many types of works that can be done with the cactus. This is just one of them.

Bamboo

Everyone nowadays knows about lucky bamboo. It is one of the easiest plants there is to grow. But what you might not know is that if you take a photo of yourself or your home and you burn it to ash, you can add that ash to the water that keeps the bamboo alive to help draw prosperity into the home. You can also feed the plant change at least once a week and say, "As I feed you, so shall you feed me." Be mindful that you are sharing your money with this plant, and you need to take good care of the plant. If the plant dies, the money dies.

Banana Tree

The banana tree is another plant that is easy to grow. It doesn't take a whole lot of maintenance other than watering it at least once a week. It can either be planted in the ground or put in a large pot. Either way they make nice plants. The banana tree is good for drawing prosperity and good spirits onto the property. These trees actually produce small bananas. The tree can be worked with for prosperity or to send an enemy down a slippery slope. Have you ever watched the cartoons of someone stepping on a banana peel and how they just take up the slide and go down. The same goes for the banana peels on the tree. I want to give you two small works: for one you will have to wait until the tree produces the baby banana, but the other one you can work with one of the leaves.

Just remember—and I cannot stress this enough—that you and only you are responsible for the works that you do. The work has to be justified or you take the chance of getting hit with your own work. When your banana tree produces clusters of small bananas, remove one of the bananas and peel it. I try to get me the banana out without pulling the whole side down on the banana. Once you have the flesh of the banana out, you will need to take a photo of your target, a foot track of the target if you can get it, red pepper, and saltpeter. Place the photo and the other ingredients inside the banana peel. Then you need some red thread to bind the banana peel closed. Once you get the peel closed, place the work out in the hot sun and let the sun do its job. If you can find the red thread after the peel disintegrates and eats through the stuff that's on the inside of it, you can take the red thread and throw it away, away from your home. Then you just sit back and wait and watch.

For this next work you need a banana leaf, a two-dollar bill, some hair off the crown of your head, and dirt from the four corners of your property and by the front door. Try to pick one of the smaller leaves. Lay the leaf out flat, place the dollar facedown on the leaf, then place the other ingredients on top of that. Take the dollar and fold it toward you with the other ingredients inside. You are making a small packet, and now fold all the banana leaf around the packet. Take some red thread and bind the packet together. You will need three sets of three seven-day candles. Place the candles in a triangle setup and put the packet in the center. Light the candles going top, left, right. Normally if you were trying to draw money, you would go from right to left, but in this instance, you're trying to grow your money so you're trying to hold on to your money. That's why you're going to go left to right. Say your prayer and your petition over the candles. Try to go daily at least three times a day to repeat your prayer and your petitions as the candles burn. Before the first set of candles burn all the way out, light your next set and just set them side by side. The candles should burn for twenty-one days. Once the twenty-one days are over, you can either put the small packet in your wallet or you can place it on a money altar if you have one. What's important is that you work that packet at least once a month.

Copper

I know copper is not a plant but it's very powerful and has strong drawing powers—particularly for prosperity. So, if you decide to do a special plant, you might consider putting it in a copper planter to make the work stronger. Some spirits have a special connection to copper. St. Peter is one of those that seems to like copper. Copper lamps and pots are powerful tools when you are doing the work. I just wanted to share this little bit of information as I have worked with copper many years.

Easter Lily

Easter lilies are very powerful plants for bringing back someone who has left. They will grow anytime, but they usually bloom during Easter. Easter, as we all know, is the time of the resurrection. I was taught that the Easter can also resurrect or revive a love that has grown cold or wandered off. You will need a new pot, potting soil, a lily, and a photo of the couple. Draw a heart around the couple and a circle around that heart. Add a layer of dirt on the bottom of the pot, then put the photo in there and add another layer of dirt. Once you have the pot set up, you can add the plant and cover the roots with the remaining soil. You need two candles: one to represent the target and one to represent the person doing the work. Set the lily in the middle of the table and place one candle each on either side of it. Say your prayer and your petition over each of the candles, and every day move the candles a little closer until they are both touching. Let the candles burn out. Once the candles have burned out, take the lily and place it on the front door stoop. Take really good care of the lily, and go daily and speak with it to pull the lover back home.

Eggs

Like copper, an egg is not plant, but you can use eggs along with plant works. Spirit cannot tell the difference between an egg and a human because they are both living things. If you are doing a work to protect anything—your home, your money, your job, whatever it may be—you can name the egg after yourself and put it in a pot with a plant of your choice. Once you get it all fixed, you can put the plant on the front door stoop somewhere in the front of the house so if anyone is throwing at you they are going to hit that egg in that plant first before they ever get you. I was taught that when you do this type of work with an egg, you clean yourself off with that egg, name the egg, and then select some ivy: these are really good for this type of work because they climb and they grow. It may seem like an easy work, but it does really well, and it will give any crossed conditions that are thrown at you somewhere else to hit.

Fern

The fern is a very powerful plant and one that can be worked with for many different types of jobs. Ferns are good for prosperity, protection, entanglement, love work, and to hide from an enemy. These are just a few things that a fern is good for. Ferns are kind of temperamental, though; they are sometimes not the easiest plant to grow. They don't like the heat, or I should say the hot sun. They need to be misted and, in my opinion, they really need to be watered at least twice a week. They need to be kept in a shaded area.

Flea Bush

There is a bush that grows wild that the old folks call flea bush. I had never heard of this bush before my husband brought it home. One summer we had fleas really bad, and we could not get rid of them—we tried everything. It seems like nothing was going to work. One of his oldest friends at work told him about flea bush. They went in the woods, and he cut a bunch of the branches and brought them home.

When he got home with the branches, I didn't know what in the world was going on. We put the branches with the leaves on them all over the house and within a day the fleas were gone. I wanted to know where I could find the plant. I asked my oldest son if he knew of the flea bush, and he said yes. He told me the real name is wax myrtle—and you're not gonna believe this—it comes from the same family as bayberry.

I wanted to share this information with y'all, because this is the type of information that is being lost as elders pass on. I tried to root the plant, but I couldn't get it to grow. It needs to be in very moist ground. Also we have to remember that whatever a plant like this does, it can also be worked with in Conjure. Since this plant gets rid of fleas, it could also be worked with to get rid of troublesome issues and folks. We have to remember that back in the day the ancestors worked with what they had, and plant knowledge is a big part of this work. It's way more than just putting conjure bags and jars together. You need to understand the elements that you're working with— what their job is, what do they do, why do we need them. Conjure always thinks of these things. Doing this work is a twenty-four hour a day, seven days a week, 365 days a year job—you have to live it. It's not just something that you do because you need something or you want something: it's a lifetime of work. If I took the work with spirits and this way of life out of my life, I would just be a shell. There would be nothing left to me because I live this work daily.

Hibiscus

Hibiscus is one of my favorite plants, and they are easy to grow. I have found that they grow better when they are planted in the east or placed in pots facing the east. They come in many different colors, but yellow and red are my favorites. I had a pair of yellow ones for years that sat on each side of my door stoop. They were fixed to draw in success and prosperity, but we had a bad flood and it killed them. So now I have red ones on either side of my door stoop in the same planters that the yellow ones lived in for so many years. The planters are made out of old tires and tire rims painted white.

I placed this particular set of planters on each side of my door stoop for a reason. Folks nowadays have lost a lot of the knowledge that their elders had. I remember growing up in the country and seeing all these old broke-down tractors and iron plows—just many different types of pieces of iron just left in the fields. One time I asked my uncle why he left the old plow in the yard.

It's not like it was there for decoration. There were no flowers planted around it, no nice flower bed or nothing: just the old plow sitting there rusted and all alone. I remember him telling me that iron keeps the witches away. He said that witches fear iron. I've never forgotten that. I truly thought that he was joking, but when I asked my aunt, she said the same thing. Only she told me that it helps protect from the blue hag and the boo hags that ride in the night. She didn't have to say anything else. I grew up on stories of boo hags and how they will slip into your room at night when you're asleep and steal your breath away. So that told me right there that the iron is something that protects.

I grew up on a lot of old stories and things that some folks call old wives' tales. These stories came from somewhere and started somewhere. And my culture is built on them, so I'm really not sure that they are stories after all.

When it comes to planting a plant for a certain condition, I always think about the job that plant has to do, and this also makes me think about the container that that plant is going to go in. I always consider all the elements and everything pertaining to the job. I'm a conjure woman twenty-four hours a day, seven days a week, 365 days a year; my whole life is built around this work. So when I am doing something for my home or for one of my clients, I always think about the condition I'm working on. The planters that my hibiscus are planted in serve a twofold purpose. For one, the iron tire rim adds protection for my door stoop, and the tire is another added protection because you can cut a tire but it takes a lot to blow one out. And then you have the red hibiscus that is planted in each one of them. I went with red this time because red is a powerful color. Red represents the blood, and it's beautiful. I didn't really do a lot to the soil that was already in the planters because that soil had already been worked for my crown of success. I just left it like it was.

I did take the soil out and clean the planter before I added my new hibiscus plants. I prayed over the soil for protection, and I put the soil and the hibiscus back in the planter. I did do one thing extra, though. Like I said, iron is very protective and very powerful. The spirits that rule iron are very powerful and very protective and dependable and unbreakable. I took two railroad spikes and fixed them for protection. Then I placed one in each of my planters so my door stoop is now double protected, and not only that, the iron will feed my hibiscus plants and make them strong.

Hibiscus is a wonderful plant because it also has healing properties. It makes a great tea. It's good for your hair. It's good for your skin. So not only is it good for protection; it's also good for health and it's a very healthy plant. It is a very beautiful plant: the flowers grow large and they are vibrant in color. The flowers can be added to healing works and other works such as love, crown of success, and prosperity. It's important for a conjure worker to look at all aspects of the plant in order to really understand how to work with that plant. Conjure work is more than meets the eye; it is about understanding nature and the things that live in it just like the ancestors of this work did.

Honeysuckle

The honeysuckle is another of my favorite plants. I remember as a child pulling the little flowers off and taking the water that was inside the flower. It's sweet. Everyone knows about the honeysuckle, but what they might not know is that the honeysuckle flowers can be worked with for long-lasting relationships for sweetening and to draw love into a relationship. You have to look at all aspects of the plant, so notice the honeysuckle grows strong and hearty and it's hard to kill them. Also the nectar is sweet, and the flowers are also beautiful. If we live by the rule of like begets like where the honeysuckle is concerned, it grow strong, will last many years, and the nectar from its flowers is sweet. If you are having issues in your relationship or if you are just beginning a new relationship with someone that you want to grow and be strong and to flourish like the honeysuckle, then this is the right plant for you to work with.

It has long been known that conjure workers work with trees. The honeysuckle is a type of tree because it grows large and thick. Here's a trick that I learned a long time ago to drop sweetness into a relationship. You are going to make a packet, so you need a small piece of cloth. A piece of the target's clothing will work best for this—unwashed if you can get it. You need three flowers from the honeysuckle and some white cotton string. Lay out the cloth and add the target's photo to it. Place the three flowers one at a time on top of the photo. You need to say your prayer and your petition over each flower before you lay it on top of the photo. You also need to petition the honeysuckle tree to help make the relationship strong, sweet, and loving.

Bind the packet up with the cotton string, remembering to say your prayer and petition over the packet as you bind it together.

Once you get the packet bound together, then you are going to tie the packet to one of the limbs of the honeysuckle. You are going to once again petition the honeysuckle to keep your relationship strong, sweet, and loving. This is not the type of work that you can just do, walk away from it, and forget about it. It is now your responsibility to make sure that that honeysuckle plant is fed, honored, and taken care of. You may be wondering how you feed the plant. You have to find the roots of the plant first. And I'm not talking about the ones that are right there at the base of the plant; you have to find the *end* of the roots. It is now your responsibility to give that plant a cool drink of water at least once a week at the root end. You can find the roots in the afternoon when the sun is high; look and see where the shadow of the plant falls. At the end of that shadow is where the roots lay, and that is where you will pour your libation for the plant once a week.

Just like when you're doing any type of plant work, if you don't take care of the plant, the work will die out. Even though the honeysuckle is a hearty plant and will continue to grow even if you don't water it, it is your responsibility to take care of that plant as that plant is working for you to help your relationship become strong and to stay sweet and loving. We have to remember that plants are living things and they have a memory and it is long. So just do the work to take care of your plant to keep your end of the bargain up.

Then stand back and watch your relationship grow strong, powerful, sweet, and loving.

Ivy

There's an old saying that love grows where ivy grows. Some folks believe that if they can't grow ivy at their home, then there is no love in that home. Ivy is one of the simplest and easiest plants to grow. It will root in water or soil, and you can grow it in your home in a large container of water. I have found that as long as you take care of the plant, it will grow. Ivy is one of the plants that I call a trailer plant because it eventually will grow running up the walls or in a window seal. It will take over a whole house if you don't keep it trimmed back. This type of plant is good for going and finding things for you like love, money, or success. They are also easy to work with, and the roots will literally grow around your petition. I've written about ivy before and working with it, but I still wanted to touch on them in this section. I'm just gonna give the layout for this type of work because it's basically the same with the petition, the only thing that changes.

I work with these plants in two different ways. One is with a cloth petition; the other is with a paper petition. I've never written about working with a cloth petition before so I'm going to give two works now: one with paper and one with cloth. Both of these works are going to be done on the vines of the ivy. This type of work is being lost in this new age.

So the first one is going to be using a strip of cloth from a target's clothing to bring them back. It doesn't have to be a large piece of cloth, and you don't have to write out a full petition. You simply have to write the target's name on the cloth and the words "come back to me." The plant is going to do the rest for you.

Once you have your cloth and you have these things written on the cloth, tape this strip of cloth and tie it on the ivy where you see the root. That is where there is a little knot on the stem of the ivy. If you broke that piece off and put it in water, it would grow. Do not tie the cloth on there too tight or you'll kill the plant, which means you'll kill the work. It just needs to be tied enough not to move up and down. As you tie the first knot, call the target's name out and petition the ivy to go get the target and bring them back. Repeat this more times to where you have a total of three knots. I like to do this type of work in the middle of the ivy to keep it away from prying eyes. Then you need to talk to the plant daily and petition the plant to bring the target back. It depends on how well you take care of the plant and the power of the target's will how long this will take. You have to remember that sometimes when you're doing this type of work, it becomes a battle of wills: who has a stronger one and who's going to give up first. Sometimes this work takes time. Our time is not Spirit's time. Just do the work and be patient.

Every one of us needs money and prosperity in our lives. There is no better way to make that happen than to work with a live plant. One of the best things about ivy plants is that they have runners, which means they grow outward and the stems multiply. It makes them wonderful plants for prosperity work. This is a simple but effective work if you need a single amount of money to pay a bill. You simply have to write it on a piece of paper and pin the petition to the ivy. Do not stick the pin in the plant itself. Fold the paper over and pin the paper where it will stay. Talk to the plants and explain the situation. Ask the plant to go and find you the money that you need to pay this bill or whatever else it is you need the money for. Remember you are dealing with a living being. They hear our petition, and if we take care of them, they take care of us. Once you get the money that you need, gently remove the petition. Burn it to ash and blow it into the east. Take care of your plants even if you are not needing them to work for you. Like I said, plants are living things, and they have a long memory.

Iron Plant

The old folks say there is power in a name, that powerful names will help you get along in life. That's why in the old days folks really thought about the names that they were giving their children. The iron plant, or cast-iron plant as some folks call it, is one of those plants that stands up to its name. These plants are almost impossible to kill. They can go without water and be left with no sun, and they will still live. Everyone knows that iron is almost invincible; cast iron is powerful, and it will last a long time. It's almost indestructible. Cast-iron skillets show us that this is true. They will last a person's lifetime and can be passed down their bloodline.

The iron plant is the perfect plant for protection work. If the plant is not able to be killed, then the work will be just as powerful. But you have to remember when you're working with live plants that if the plant dies, the work dies plain and simple. The work cannot live on without the plant.

When I fix these plants for family members or clients, I like to have a photo of the house. If the house is protected, the folks inside the house are going to be protected. I also take the dirt from the four corners of the property, so the property will also be protected. If you have need of this work, you need to get an iron plant, a nice pot to put it in, a photo of the house or you can even do a family photo, and the dirt from the four corners of the land.

Spiritually cleanse the pot, and then mix the soil with the dirt from the four corners of the property. Add a little bit of dirt to the pot, then place the photo that you have written your petition on inside the pot. Cover the photo with a little bit of potting soil, then you add your plant. Fill the pot the rest of the way with the soil so that the base of the plant is covered. Once you have the plant settled in, put the plant in a window facing the east where the front door of your home should be. Make sure that you take very good care of this plant, and it will take care of you and your family.

There's also a little trick that I learned from one of my elders working with this plant for protection of your money. Make a packet with your photo and the hair from the crown of your head out of a two-dollar bill. Then you plant the two-dollar-bill packet in a pot with the plant covering the packet. You put the plant directly on top of the packet with no pot and soil in between the packet and the plant roots. You want the roots to grow around the packet. You petition the plant to protect your money. Remember as the plant grows, your money will grow as long as you take care of that plant. This work is not a get rich fast type of work. Plants grow slowly. They have to be fed and taken care of. So take care of the plant and let it do its job.

Jalapeño

Jalapeño plants are great for doing shut your mouth work and for heating up a target's head. Sometimes you don't have to work against the target; you simply have to make them hotheaded enough so that they show who they really are. There are a lot of folks who hide their true selves behind a mask. These folks are masters at playing the game. Folks don't usually realize who they really are until it's too late and they are in too deep with the target.

When you work with a jalapeño plant, it's like a double-edged sword: it hits the target twice especially if you eat the jalapeños. When you eat a jalapeño, it goes in one way and comes out another; this is some of the strongest work that you can do against a target. I'm not going to just come out and say what I'm talking about. I am a lady after all. You're going to have to read behind the lines and understand what I'm saying.

The thing to remember when working with a jalapeño plant is that even the roots and the dirt that that plant is growing in pick up the heat from the plant. This is one reason that if you're going to be a conjure worker you really need to learn about plants and the fruits and flowers that they put out. I keep saying this over and over again, and I know folks get tired of it, but there's more to this work than what most folks realize. Ancestors couldn't run to the grocery store and buy all these pre-ready roots and herbs and all these things that New Age workers work with nowadays. They had to work with what they had. This means that they had to know the land and the plants that grew on that land and how those dirts and plants could be worked with. If you're going to be a real traditional conjure worker, then you need to get out of this box that most young workers without a mentor or a teacher are in. You are boxing yourself in to only learn a little bit of this work when there is so much more to it. You know I've made some folks mad because I write and they feel like I'm telling too much, and yet some of these same folks don't believe that I should be able to do this work. If I don't share the work, then the work is going to be lost. And no one is going to have it because some of the same folks are in that box and all they know is what they have read about when this work is so much more.

I want to talk about the roots of the jalapeño plant before I go along and finish talking about helping a target show their true colors. If you have a jalapeño or any type of hot pepper plant that has died for whatever reason, don't throw the roots away. You can work with those roots. All you have to do is pull the roots up and trim the dead part off of the roots so it's manageable. Now you have a working tool that you can use to do shut your mouth type work. Simply hang the roots up somewhere, and when you have a situation when you need to shut someone up, you can simply insert their photo in the roots of that hot pepper plant and go through the petitions and the prayers. The root will last you a lifetime. Once you achieve the goal that you had for that target, you simply remove the paper, burn it to ash, and blow it into the west to keep it away from you. I just wanted to share that old work with you, and there's many more like that. I'm getting older, and if I don't share these works and other elders are not sharing works like they used to, eventually there's not going to be any more knowledge shared. Then all you're going to have is what you can find on the internet or what folks have written about.

Now back to making a target show their true self. This works really well because when folks are hotheaded, they act without thinking. And if you act without thinking, then you are showing who you truly are. Take the target's photo and wrap it around the roots of a new jalapeño plant. You can pin it on the roots using two needles that you have cut the eyes off of. You will run one needle going one way and the other needle crossing it where it looks like a cross to hold the photo on to the section of the roots. Then you plant the jalapeño plant. You name the plant after the target, and as the plant grows, the heat of the peppers will grow. They will get hotter and hotter. As the jalapeños mature, that heat gets stronger and so will the work. You will notice that the target is beginning to become confused and very hotheaded. Their guard will be down, and folks will begin to see exactly who and what they are.

This is not the type of work that you would do on someone just because they made you mad. You have to remember that every action causes a reaction and we are responsible for all of our actions. This is definitely a work that you should do divination on before you put it in motion. You are taking on the responsibility to bring forth justice against the target, so make sure you have the right to do so and your own plate is clean.

Joshua Tree

I have been drawn to the Joshua trees since I first saw them about twelve years ago on a trip to Santa Cruz, California. I was going there to teach at the Serpent's Kiss. I was with my daughter, and we were driving from Texas to California. Somehow, we took a wrong turn and ended up where the Joshua trees grow. It reminded me of the book of Joshua in the Bible, especially Joshua at the walls of Jericho. I remember we stopped to get gas, and inside the gas station they were selling Joshua tree seeds. I remember the lady telling us that it was against the law to dig up a small Joshua tree. The only way you can have a tree is either to plant it by the seeds or buy one, and you must have the paperwork to show that you bought the tree legally. I was infatuated by those trees. They look like arms raised up to the heavens.

I bought a pack of the seeds, but I have never planted them. If I can find a pack of seeds, I put them up to keep them safe, which is something I do all the time and end up misplacing whatever it is I put up. The Joshua tree is not really a tree; it is a yucca plant. When I got back home, I went to see one of my elders and asked her if she had ever heard of a Joshua tree. I had tried to research about it, but I couldn't find anything. She told me that the tree is named after Joshua because God gave Joshua a power that the Bible says equaled Moses's power. She told me that there is an old tale about Joshua while going to battle for God. This battle can be found in the book of Joshua chapter 8. It said that the arms of the Joshua tree represent the arms that Joshua raised up to heaven calling on God. I have asked other elders, and although they didn't go into detail, they all agreed that the Joshua tree was named after the prophet Joshua and that it stands tall just as Joshua did.

I've added Joshua 8 V 30–35 here where it tells of Joshua after a battle building an altar to the Lord as God had commanded. The Joshua tree is very powerful, so I just want to add it to this book to share the knowledge my elder had shared with me. It seems like this knowledge of the Joshua tree is being lost.

> *30 Now Joshua built an altar to the Lord God of Israel in Mount E'bal,*
>
> *31 As Moses the servant of the Lord had commanded the children of Israel, as it is written in the Book of the Law of Moses: "an altar of whole stones over which no man has wielded an iron tool." And they offered on it burnt offerings to the Lord, and sacrificed peace offerings.*
>
> *32 And there, in the presence of the children of Israel, he wrote on the stones a copy of the law of Moses, which he had written.*

33 Then all Israel, with their elders and officers and judges, stood on either side of the ark before the priests, the Levites, who bore the ark of the covenant of the Lord, the stranger as well as he who was born among them. Half of them were in front of Mount Gerizim and half of them in front of Mount Ebal, as Moses the servant of the Lord had commanded before, that they should bless the people of Israel.

34 And afterward he read all the words of the law, the blessings and the cursings, according to all that is written in the Book of the Law.

35 There was not a word of all that Moses had commanded which Joshua did not read before all the assembly of Israel, with the women, the little ones, and the strangers who were living among them.

Lemon/Lime

I started to leave the lemons and limes out of this section, but then I decided that folks really don't understand how they work. They are kind of like a double-edged sword because they can be worked with to sour a target but also for cleansings in bitter baths. They are both very powerful when it comes to cut and clear works. Both of them will strip away a cross condition, and they are good for your hair and your skin. On the other hand, they can be worked with to sour a target's life. It really all depends on the job.

If you work with them for cleansing, you have to be mindful that they strip away everything—the good and the bad. So once you're through with the cleansing, you have to replace what you took off. If you do what is called a bitter bath, then you need to follow up with a sweetening bath. I will usually do three bitter baths in a row, wait a day, and follow up with three sweetening baths. When I say three baths, I don't mean three in the same day. There are actually some folks that would not understand that I mean three baths on three consecutive days, so I just want to make that clear. I would also like to caution you about cleansing your head with either one of these fruits because they do strip away everything. Always protect the crown of your head.

I'm going to give you a work for souring a target should the need ever arise. I once had someone ask me if I really have done all the works that I write about. The answer is yes. I have been doing this work since I was seventeen years old. I'm way in my middle sixties now, so yes, if I write about it, I've done it. There is a simple way that you can sour a target and move them out of the way, but remember you and you alone are responsible for the works that you do. No one else is responsible—only you—and all works of this type should only be done if they are justified. You should always do divination before you do this type of work; if the work is not justified, it can be reversed and you will be hit with your own work.

To do this work, you need a lemon or a lime, four needles, three stick candles, some black cotton thread, and a rock from a train track. You also need a photo or the name of the target. Cut the lemon or lime in half. And in one half stick the photo of the target, and in the other half put the rock from the train track. Mash them down in the center of the lemon or lime. Put the two halves together, and insert the four needles in the shape of a cross to hold the work together. Take the black thread and wrap it going away from you while calling out the target's name and saying your petition. Make sure that the work is covered with the black thread. Once this is done, place one of the stick candles on top of the work. Light the candle and say your prayer and petition at least three times while the hands of the clock are going downward. That means only start when the hands are at five after the hour. Burn a candle on the work three days in a row. On the fourth day take the lime or lemon and go throw it on the railroad track. This work not only sours your target but also removes them from you.

As a side note, be very careful burning the candle on the work. You have to watch it closely and put the candle out before the fire reaches the thread. Please use caution when you are burning candles and when you are doing this type of work. Never leave candles unattended.

Morning Glory

Old folks say that the morning glory draws in the glory and the blessings of God. The plant keeps God's hand on the property. Morning glories climb, so they are a great plant to send to find the blessings you are looking for. They are also a favored plant for hummingbirds. Hummingbirds not only bring in blessings, but they also take the messages you are petitioning for out into the world. Morning glories should be planted in the east where the sun rises, although they can grow in shaded areas. Placing them in the east pulls down the sun's energy and power into the vines, which in turn empowers the plant.

Morning glories can be planted in large pots or in hanging baskets that can be hung on either side of the doorway. This is definitely one of the plants you need planted close to the front doorway or front gate. Remember any plant that you work for magic needs to be well taken care of. If the plant dies, the magic dies with it. Working a plant for magic is called tricking or conjuring the plant. In this day and time most folks would call it putting a spell on the plant.

If you decide to work a morning glory for prosperity, you need a clean flowerpot that you have spiritually cleansed with the wash of your choosing. You need a few scoops of dirt from each side of the door stoop from your front and back door. You will need a good type of potting soil and a petition written out along with Psalm 23. You will mix the dirt from your front and back door with the potting soil. Place a thin layer of potting soil in the bottom of your container, say your prayer and petition over the potting soil, then place your petition and the Psalm 23 on top of the soil. Then you add another small layer of dirt and transplant the morning glory into the new pot. Once you have the morning glory planted, then once again you say your prayer and your petition along with the Psalm 23 over the plant three times. Give the plant a good drink of water. Place the plant in the east where the sun rises. Make sure to water the plant once a week and to repeat your prayer and petition along with Psalm 23 over the plant three times. It's important that you do this when you water your plant because not only are you giving the plant water, you're also feeding the plant with your prayers and the Psalm 23.

Moss

Moss is one of my favorite things to work with. It is good for entanglements, bindings, protections, and hiding things. In order to work with plants, you need to look at them and see how they grow, what the flowers look like, and how they feel when you touch them. Keep that in mind and think about moss: it looks like just one big tangled web. Not only does it look like a tangled web; it has things hidden within it like chiggers and other little bugs that you never see. Not only does it have things hidden within it; it also catches things. So because things can hide within it and it catches sticks and leaves and things that fall out of the trees, it is good for protection, for binding, and for holding things in place.

The thing that I think that most folks don't understand is that moss is an air plant. As long as you keep it misted, it will grow. Some folks believe that it will suffocate a tree, but this is not true.

We all need protection in this day and age. Too many folks know how to do this work, and some of them have no ethics. I know I'm repeating myself, but it's important that you understand that every work that you do you are responsible for. I'm going to give you two simple works that you can do working with moss. We have to remember that the ancestors of this work didn't have a whole lot of ingredients; they couldn't run to the store to get a bag full of things to do a job. They had to work with what they had. Sometimes this work seems too simple to be true, but these works come from a time when there was a need for survival and they are indeed powerful.

Protection Work with Moss

The first work I am going to share with you is a work for protection. You need some red flannel—just a small square—your photographs, a little bit of hair from the crown of your head, some red cotton thread, and some moss. You are going to make a protection packet. You will need a verse out of the Bible: 2 Timothy 4 V 18. You can either tear it directly out of the Bible or you can print it out. A trick that I have learned is when I am putting Bible verses over photos,

I will print the photo out and then print the Bible verse out on top of the photo, especially when I'm doing protection work, or you can just place the verse on top of the photo. Take the red flannel square and place the photo in the center of it. Then place the Bible verse on top of the photo and your hair on top of the Bible verse. Then place a small bit of cotton over all the ingredients. Pray that 2 Timothy 4 V 18 over the work three times and say your petition for protection over the work three times. Once this is done, fold the flannel into a small packet and use the thread to bind the packet together. Once this is done, take a tealight and set it on top of the packet. Light the tealight and repeat the prayer and petition three times over the packet as the tealight burns. Once the tealight burns out, remove the tin off the packet—be careful because those little tins get really hot and that's why they work so well. Wrap the packet with moss, covering it well where you can't see what is inside the moss.

> *And the Lord shall deliver me from every evil work,*
> *and will preserve me unto his heavenly kingdom:*
> *to whom be glory for ever and ever. Amen.*

Once you have the packet completely covered, then you will set it in a triangle setup of tealights. The tealights should be set down top, left, and then right. You light the tealights in the order that you set them down. Say your prayer and your petition over the tealights as they burn. You will need to do this setup for seven days. Once the seven days are over with, you take your packet and put it in a safe place. Once a month you can feed the packet either protection oil or olive oil you have prayed Psalm 23 into.

To Bind an Enemy with Moss

This work is to bind someone who is causing you or a loved one harm. Once again, this type of work should never be done without divination first. We don't never know what Spirit's actions are going to be toward the target. Sometimes you won't need to do anything because Spirit is already taking care of the issue. We have to remember that our time is not always Spirit's time. This is why it is important to do divination before you start this type of work. Discernment is a must when you are going against someone. I had an issue that I really wanted to work, but when I went to my spirits, they told me not to lift a hand toward this target that they were handling it. Patience is not one of my virtues, but I listened to them and in the end they have done more harm to this target than I could have ever had the heart to do. You have to always remember that any works that you do against someone should always be justified, and divination is how you find out.

For this work you need red flannel, black cotton string, moss, dirt from a jailhouse, a photo or the name of the target. You also need Deuteronomy 28 V 7. Lay the flannel out just like you did in the protection work above. Then place the photo, then the prayer, and then the dirt from the jailhouse on top of it. Fold the red flannel into a packet while you pray the prayer and your petition, bind the packet with the black cotton string, then cover the packet with the moss. Bind the moss with more of the black cotton string while you are saying the prayer and your petition. Once you have the packet put together, set it up in a cross setup with black seven-day candles. The setup is placed top, bottom, left, right, and the packet is set in the center. Light the candles in the way that you set them up. Say your prayer and petition over the setup three times and then three times a day until the setup has burned out. You can either keep the packet and continue to work it or take the packet to stagnant water and throw it in. I leave that up to you.

> *The LORD shall cause thine enemies that rise up against thee to be smitten before thy face: they shall come out against thee one way, and flee before thee seven ways.*

Mother-in-Law's Tongue

The mother-in-law's tongue, or snake plant as some folks call it, is well-known by the elders to keep gossip and nosy neighbors away from the house. This plant should be planted by the front door or an entrance door where folks come in and out of the home. This plant also protects the home. St. Ramon is the owner of this plant. He is well-known for shutting down gossip and backbiting. St. Ramon is a saint of justice.

If you are having issues with folks who gossip about you or your family or if you are having issues within the home with too much arguing, this plant is the perfect one to have in the home and outside the door where folks come into the home. You will need a new pot that has been spiritually cleansed, potting soil, the plant, and a St. Ramon novena. Write your petition on the novena. Place a thin layer of potting soil in the pot, then place the novena that you have written your petition on on top of the potting soil, then place another thin layer of potting soil over the novena.

Hold the roots of the plant in your hand and pray St. Ramon's novena over the roots three times. Petition St. Ramon to stop all gossip and all troubles within your home, then place the roots gently in the pot and cover them with potting soil. Give the plant a good drink of water and repeat the novena and your petition over the plant. Water your plant once a week, and make sure to say your prayer and petition along with the novena over the plant after you water it. This should keep all those wagging tongues at bay.

Oak

The oak is a very powerful tree. We have two very large ones on our property: one at the front on the north side by the crossroads and the other one on the other side of the property on the south side. Normally I would say that things don't grow on the north side very well, but the oak tree there is an old tree and it's been there a long time. I've lived in this house for thirty-four years and that tree was there when we moved here. It almost seems like it stands guard over our property. The other oak tree on the south side of the property is also a huge tree and it's all been here a longer time—the one on the north side is the younger of the two.

Those trees have withstood numerous hurricanes and blood storms, and they're still standing strong. The oak tree is known for its strength. If you needed to stop someone and you needed the power to do it, you could nail their photo facing inward on an oak tree and petition that tree to give you the power to stop that target. Oaks also offer protection and prosperity. If you can find an acorn from an old tree, those are very lucky if carried in your pocket to draw forth prosperity and success. Oak trees are one of the trees that should never be cut down as they hold the wisdom of the elders. They also have healing properties to them. If you have an oak on your land or near your property, take good care of it and cherish it.

Okra

Okra is a very powerful plant! Not only is it healthy for you to eat, but it is also a great spiritual cleanser. The ancestors brought okra seeds over on the slave ships in their hair. Once they got here and got settled, they planted the seeds. Now okra is a staple of folks in the South. The only drawback from okra is a slime that comes from it, but that is actually what does the cleansing. I was taught that an okra bath is taken cold. This is one of the strongest cleansing baths that I know of. Get you a dishpan and put some cool water in it. Cut up about seven okra pods in little round circles and place these in the water to make the wash.

I like to set a white candle in the wash. I will place a small can in the wash and set the candle in it. While the candle burns, I will move the okra around in the opposite direction of the hands of the clock with my hand, praying that whatever is on me be removed and reversed. I will repeat the prayers off and on until the candle goes out. I remove the tin can, and then using my hand, I will go in the opposite direction of the clock three times while asking that whatever is there be removed and returned. And then I will go in the direction of the hands of the clock and ask that protection and blessings be brought in.

Once this is done, I will remove all of the plant material out of the water and I'll squeeze it so I can get all of the slime out of it. Those okra seeds could be planted, and then you can grow your own okra. Okra is easy to grow in the sun if you keep it watered well. Now that my bath is ready, I wait for the hands of the clock to reach five after the hour, and then I'll go take my bath. I take a shower first to clean my body and then I pour the wash over my head using a cup to make sure that I get the full effect of the wash. I leave the slime on me for about five minutes as I pray for cleansings and blessings.

This is a very strong way to do cleansing work, so I wouldn't do more than three baths in a row once a month at the most. You won't want to do too many cleansing baths, or you will wash away your good luck along with the bad.

Petunias

Petunias are good to hang at the door or around the front door for protection. The red and purple ones are the strongest ones. We all know that red is a powerful color as it represents the blood. It's a hot color and it also draws. Purple is also a powerful color that can dominate. It can represent success and also royalty. Petunias are good to hang by the door because they have a sticky film on them, and this will help catch anything that is thrown at you or your home. If you want to hang a set of petunias on each side of the door in a hanging basket, then you need to take a photo of your home, write your petition over the photo, and then plant the photo in each hanging basket or pot while you petition the spirit and the life of that plant to catch anything that's thrown at your home. Make sure you water the plant well and take care of it, and the plant will take care of you.

Peace Lily

When we first moved into this house, there was a flower bed that ran the whole length of the front of the house. Even though it was grown over, you could still see the peace lilies with their beautiful white flowers. I remember getting out there on my knees and pulling up all the weeds and grass that had grown around that area, but somehow those peace lilies lived through all of that. They lived for a long time, and then we had a bad hurricane and they never came back. Every year they would come back in the same place, and then they didn't.

When we first moved here, I wasn't sure what those flowers were until Meme, one of my elders, came one day and told me they were peace lilies and would bring peace to the home. She told me that you could take three of the flowers and place of photo of the family in the three flowers and bind them together with red cotton string. And then you hang that packet over the front door to ensure that the home would always be peaceful. Peace lilies are very easy to grow. You can even grow them inside the house in a sunny window in a pot, and they will give the home a peaceful faith.

Pine

Pine puts off a sap that's very, very sticky. This sap is good for a few things; it can be healing, but it can also hold things together. If you are having trouble keeping your man at home, you can take a photo of the inside of the house and a photo of him and get you some kind of sap that is sticky. Smear this on the photo of the inside of the house and then put his photo on top of the sap. You kind of mash them together and they'll stay stuck. Every man has his favorite chair in the house to sit in; most of the time it's a recliner. You are going to plant this simple little trick under the seat of his recliner. You simply have to flip the recliner over and put the packet between the springs of the seat. By doing this you will stick his butt to that seat, which means his rambling and moving around should slow down. Don't let the simplicity of this trick fool you: sometimes simple tricks are the best.

Pomegranate Tree

There are many plants that belong to many different spirits, and this is one of the plants that belong to St. Peter. St. Peter loves the pomegranate tree. I have two of them out in the garden, one on each side of the doorway. As we know from the Bible, St. Peter holds the keys to the door and to the gates and to the roads. Both of those trees are dedicated to St. Peter. When I feed the trees, I'm also feeding St. Peter. As we know, trees and plants are living things and they have their own spirit to them. Some of them are very protective, some of them draw in prosperity, and some of them, like the pomegranate tree, open the way. Mine are miniature pomegranates, which you can grow in large pots.

If you are drawn to work with St. Peter, you can buy you a miniature pomegranate tree, place it in a nice pot at the front door on the left-hand side, and dedicate it to St. Peter. Petition St. Peter and tell him that you are giving him the tree and ask him to make the tree protect your home, keep your roads open, and keep you well protected in the name of St. Peter. Make sure you take care of that tree. That is the place you go to give your petitions to St. Peter because once you dedicate the tree to him, that tree belongs to him.

Shame Plant

The shame plant is very easy to grow. It doesn't take a lot to take care of it. The old folks will tell you that a name holds power and the names of flowers, fruits, and vegetables give you the idea of what you can work with those items. So the shame plant can be worked with to draw shame upon a transgressor. There's a lot of times when folks nowadays think that they can just do whatever they want and treat folks any way they want to. And they get away with it because folks don't see the real them. If you want to bring attention to someone who needs to be shamed, you take their photo and you write their transgression across the photo. Then you plant it with the shame plant. You need to feed and water that plant and treat the plant well. Every time you feed and water the plant, you repeat your petition of what needs to be done. Before you realize what is happening, you will start hearing little things about the transgressor. Folks will start noticing the wrongs that they're doing until eventually they are totally out in the open and everyone sees them for exactly who and what they are. These works don't work overnight. You have to be patient and you have to be diligent with your prayers and your petition, but as the plant grows, your work should grow.

Sunflower

When my grandchildren were small, every year we would plant sunflowers out by the fence. There would be a whole line of sunflowers out there. They would get out there in the dirt and count the seeds, and we would all plant a seed with a blessing on it. We did this every year, and we always had the most beautiful sunflowers you have ever seen. I miss those times, but they're all grown now and all have their own lives. They don't have time to come around to plant sunflowers anymore, but they will always have that memory. Sunflowers planted in the east bring forth prosperity, happiness, and success. These are all things that the flowers themselves are known for within magic. Just think of the magic that you would have if you had a pot of sunflowers sitting at the front of your house next to your front door. The sunflower also brings forth happiness—just looking at them makes you feel good.

I tried to plant sunflowers every year in a pot by the front door. I have some large pots that I put these types of plants in. And every year I will write my petition out and plant it in the potting soil before I plant the seed. The flowers will grow perfectly fine in a good pot with good soil it. You could plant them in the front of the house to draw in all of the magic that the sunflowers are known for.

Sweet Potato

Sweet potatoes are very good for drawing in prosperity and money. I keep one growing here on the windowsill. To fix a sweet potato, you need a large jar, three toothpicks, the sweet potato, and your petition. Cleanse the jar well and then stick three toothpicks into the sweet potato and set that to the side. Take your petition and burn it to ash. Put the ash into the jar, and fill the jar with water. Then take the sweet potato and set it on top of the jar. You need to make sure that the potato is not touching the water. As the potato grows, vines will start coming out of the potato. These vines are what is going to go find you your money, prosperity, and success. If you need a certain amount of money, write it down and fix it on one of the vines. Once the money comes, remove the petition, burn it to ash, and blow it to the east. These sweet potatoes will last forever. I had one for about eight years, and then I don't know what happened but it just died. It became too soft. So I've started another one. This is the easy way to do prosperity work out in the open, and folks won't even realize what you're doing. So this truly is a trick.

Thorny Plants

Thorny plants are one of the best protections that you can have growing around your house—especially the thorny vines that run along the fence. We have a large one out in front of my house, and in the summertime that thing grows huge and will run along the fence line. And we have roses planted out there in the front also for protection. My mama used to have rosebushes in the front of the house in front of the windows. I didn't think about it at the time, being a kid, but I now know that those were there for protection. It takes a lot to get through a thorny bush. This is one of the reasons that cacti are so protective: those thorns will draw blood.

So, for those who might not really understand how the plants work and what they do, the idea behind plants with thorns or plants that have runners on them or plants like moss is that they entangle the work. Here's an example for you. Let's say someone was throwing at you and you had all these beautiful plants in front of your home that had thorns on them, like rosebushes or big cacti on either side of your door. The old folks teach us that it would be hard for the work to get through because the thorns on the bush or the cacti would cut the work up. If you have vines that have thorns on them, that's even better because the work has to get through the vines first, and by the time the work gets through the vines, the thorns have already cut it up so that it goes nowhere. So it's always good to have some type of plant that has thorns on it somewhere in the front of your home to offer you protection.

Weeping Willow Tree

The weeping willow is one of my favorite trees. The old folks say that whatever is planted under the willow tree will shed many a tear. The long strands that shape the willow tree are great for doing binding work. They will bend, and you can literally tie one in a knot. If you have someone that has done you wrong and you are seeking justice, you can get a limb off of the weeping willow tree to bind them with. You make a regular packet on the target, then you take the limb and you wrap it around that packet. Once you get the packet fixed, then you make three knots tying the packet off. You may think that it's not possible to be able to wrap or tie anything with the limb, but you simply have to get the piece of the limb that is hanging down close to the ground.

I have to tell this story. One time I needed some weeping willow, and the only tree that we could find was in someone's yard. It was me, my daughter, and Shan. My daughter was like, "Mom, I am not going in someone's yard and these folks have a dog!" I was like, "That little doggie ain't gonna hurt you. I need a willow cutting." She was adamant she was not going to go. Then good old Shan said, "Mama, I'll go out and get it. How much do you need?" I said, "I just need a few pieces. So I'll show you." And we pulled over. We didn't see anybody and no dog. Everything looked really good. Shan got out and got to the tree. She cut the pieces I needed, and then guess what? Yeah, here came that little dog just a running just as fast as his little legs would carry him and having a meltdown. Needless to say, Shan got my weeping willow and got back into the car safe before the little monster dog could get her.

I could have gone to an old tree that I've been going to for forty years, but I needed the cuttings off this tree because this tree sat at a crossroads. It sits at a four-way stop, and since I was doing a job where I needed to put a stop to something, I needed the cuttings from that exact tree. Being a conjure woman ain't always easy. Sometimes you've got to go out at night. And sometimes you got the brave little dogs. Sometimes you have to go where you shouldn't be. But it's all in a day's work to fill the commitment that I made to my community.

Witch Hazel

I wanted to add witch hazel here because this is what my mother had us clean our faces with when we were growing up. My skin always looked good and felt good. I just simply wanted to put this here because I know nowadays a lot of folks have issues with their skin and blemishes. I don't know if it's the chemicals that are in the water nowadays or just around in general that are making folks' skin break out. Witch hazel is good. I still clean my face with it every morning. They say old habits die hard, and that's one I'm not ever going to grow out of, I guess. It's also good for bugbites and mosquito bites. It's an astringent so it pulls out whatever those little bugs leave when they bite you.

Planting the Seeds

I grew up on the old saying that if you plant the seed, the tree will grow. This was a lesson from more than one of my elders, and they were not necessarily talking about seeds for plants and fruits. They were talking about the seeds that we plant in our daily lives: every action causes a reaction and everything that we do takes seed. This was a lesson for me to learn in life and in Conjure. Sometimes when you are doing a work against a target, you just have to plant the seed that the work is being done. Then the tree will grow.

So when you're doing this type of work, every seed that you plant is important. That's why working with houseplants is so powerful—or with any plant including the ones that are outside.

It's all about the prayer and the petition that you put into the roots of that plant. If you are going to start a plant from seed, then you need to work the seeds before you plant them. And by this I mean you need to set the seeds in the center of a candle setup and say your petition and your prayer over those seeds for at least seven to nine days before you plant them. It doesn't matter what type of setup you use. It can either be a triangle, a cross, or a circle setup: any of these will work. What's important is that you do the work and you say your prayers and petition over the seeds.

If you're going to do some type of protection work for your home, then that is what you will pray over the seeds. If you are going to do some type of prosperity work, then that will be your prayer and your petition. It all depends on what it is that you are trying to achieve with the plant.

The main thing that you need to remember is that once you put the seed in the soil, you still have to continue to work over the seedlings. You can't just put the seeds in the soil and then forget about it. You have to continue going and saying your prayers and your petitions over those seedlings every day and even after they've sprouted until they get them growing really well.

Once they can be transplanted into another container and they're large enough, then you won't have to say your prayer and petition over them every day anymore. You can just go to once a week for the prayers and petitions. But remember: Like everything, a plant is a living thing. You have to take care of it. You have to feed it and water it. And if it's a magical plant, you have to understand if the plant dies, the magic dies also. Conjure is called work for a reason: it takes a lot of work to be successful. You can do it! You just have to put in the time to prosper from your efforts.

Cuttings and Roots

Our elders and ancestors knew when the time was right to plant, to pull weeds, and to gather plants. That knowledge is being lost today, so I want to add some of that information here. This is knowledge that you don't hardly ever read about, if at all. I feel like if you are going to be any type of worker of plants, herbs, trees, and the land, then you need to at least know the basics of when it is time to plant, time to gather, and time to work with these plants.

I was taught that all plants come under two categories: one is hot and sweet, and the other one is cold and bitter. These types of plants are gathered at two separate times of the day. It depends on what category they fall in as to if they are hot and sweet or cold and bitter.

Planting and growing also have times of day when they should be attended to. If you plant a plant when the sun is going down, that plant is going to struggle to grow. I'm not saying that it won't grow, but you are going to have a harder time keeping it alive. The only time that I would plant a plant when the sun is going down is if it is a loaded plant when I am doing a work on the target to slow them down. Then I would plant that plant with the sun going down, because while the plant is struggling, the target will begin to struggle. Any other time, though, I try to do my planting in the morning when the sun is high in the sky. This seems to be a good time to plant, and those plants seem to flourish.

So here are a few little things that I grew up hearing and that I follow: Never gather plants in the afternoon. Never gather plants when the sun is going down—unless it's a bitter plant. Plant on the full moon at sunrise. The roots and bark are gathered at different times of the day. Roots should be gathered before the sun sets on the bitter plant; plants should be gathered as the sun is rising on the sweet plant. Bark is gathered at the tree after the sun sets. My mama told me that when you trim the bark off of a tree when the sun is high, it pulls the life juice out of the tree and it takes a while for the tree to heal the place where you pulled the bark or the sap. But if you do it after the sun starts to go down, the tree heals itself faster. I would think that it would heal itself slower because the sun is going down, but I saw my mama take sap for healing and we would stand there until the sap stopped dripping.

I've already talked about hot and cold, sweet and bitter roots and herbs earlier in this book, but I just want to touch on them again here. Lavender is considered a sweet herb, but it could also be considered a hot and cold herb. That may sound kind of confusing, but it is really not when you look at how lavender works when it is worked with. If you have a headache and you smell fresh lavender, it has a sweet cool smell to it that almost instantly lifts the headache. But depending on the work that you are doing, lavender can also bring forth heat. It all depends on the work and your prayer and petitions, which reinforce that root or plant or tree bark or whatever you're working on.

The weeping willow tree would be considered a bitter tree. If you were going to collect the leaves or a switch off that tree for work, you would do it when the sun is going down. Growing up, I was taught not to play around with the weeping willow tree. My grandma used to say whoever sits down under that tree will weep in numbers of three. The weeping willow tree is a dominating tree. It is worked with by old-timey conjure workers to whip their enemies into shape; it is also worked to bring forth tears. The weeping willow tree can also dry tears, as we saw. It really depends on the worker and their intentions toward the target. This is the one of those trees that brings to mind what I've said before: You and you alone are responsible for the work that you do. Just because you have knowledge of something, that does not mean that you have to put that knowledge to work. You should always do a divination really before you do any type of work with a tree like the willow. Just be mindful of your actions and remember every action causes a reaction.

Woods to Keep in Mind

ANCESTOR TREE: The leaves of the ancestor tree can be worked with when doing works dealing with anything to do with the ancestors. You can wrap the leaves around a petition and wrap it in a white cloth, then bind the cloth with red cotton string tying three knots.

APPLE: Good for wisdom, prosperity, and love.

CHERRY BARK: This can be worked for all matters of love and attraction. It is said to bring forth that primal sexual attraction.

COTTON: Good to work with in protection works, defense works, and blessing works.

HOLLY: The holly tree is well known for protection. The leaves of the tree have sharp points that can draw blood. The trees are usually planted on each side of an entrance to protect the folks inside the building. This keeps the good helpful spirits in and the dark ones out.

LIGHTNING STRUCK WOOD: Adds power to any type work, but it works really well with commanding, courage, love, blockbuster, or success work.

OAK: Used for power and protection. It also removes crossed conditions.

OLIVE: This biblical tree is used for blessing and protection; you can make an all-purpose dressing oil by adding olive leaves to oil. Add the leaves to any peaceful home or peaceful works.

ORANGE: Work with to draw and all attraction work.

PALO SANTO: Adding this for my daughter who loves this stuff! Not traditionally used in Conjure work, but it is good for cleansings and healing work.

PINE: Good for healing works and for sealing things or folks off; pine sap closes things.

PEACH: Worked with for all love and sweet works.

TOBACCO LEAVES AND SUCKERS: Tobacco leaves are good to wrap work in and as the leaf dries the work gets stronger. The sucker does just as the name implies; if it isn't removed from the plant, it will suck the life out of it.

CURING CONJURE: HERBAL REMEDIES

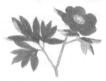

I want to share some of my family's and elders' herbal remedies that have been passed down to me. I thought it was important for folks to understand that doctoring and Conjure go hand in hand. The ancestors believed that in order for a root doctor to be successful, they had to be able to work with both hands; in other words be a two-handed worker who could both heal and hurt. If you couldn't do both, you weren't worth much.

I really don't like it when folks act like they have a big secret that no one else knows. The remedies and the foods that go with this culture and work are part of Conjure. It all went hand in hand. But when the great hoodoo highway opened on the internet and that first website and online class started, they only had a small piece of what books said Conjure was, and it shows in every one of their students 'cause they all spout the same information.

There were no real doctors for the slaves; they tended to their own with the knowledge they had of roots and herbs from their homelands. Even though the vegetation was different, they learned the power in the roots, herbs, and trees around them. They knew just the right doses and when to give them. They knew what time of day to gather what they needed. They knew in what directions the plant should face and what part of the plant was needed.

My mama grew up learning this knowledge. She treated us with all kinds of concoctions, and they worked. I have never really written about this at length. I've only hinted at it in my other writings. The old-time remedies are just as large a part of this work as the work part is. I think that it is time for folks to really see and understand what the work really is. I'm sure some won't like it and others will be pissed because I am giving away secrets, but I'm tired of all this whitewashing mixing and moxing that has gone on for the last ten years on the internet.

The thing is that the knowledge out there online is only half of it, and folks are filling books with that information. You cannot remove parts of this work to suit you or your spiritual path. There are prayers and things that go along with these healing works. This is where the remedies and Conjure walk hand in hand: someone is tricked and the worker takes it off.

I'm just tired of some folks acting like they are big hand workers or they have this great secret that only a few chosen folks know. I was raised on these remedies, but for a long time I just didn't want the fight that sharing this information is gonna cause, because with this information other folks will be able to put the puzzle together and the world might be blessed with a few well-rounded workers who can not only talk the talk but walk the walk. I have sat back worrying about folks' feelings and such till I'm wore out: no more talking around this work or just not sharing things folks need to know. I hope you enjoy this section of the book.

The Ingredients of Conjure

You may say: "I already know conjure work!" But you don't, not really—unless you have had an elder who is teaching you. This information wasn't out there, and it is only just starting to filter out now 'cause folks just can't leave things hidden. They have gathered this information from old writings and journals they have dug through for information. Doctoring folks who are ailing with the roots, herbs, trees, and whatever else is needed covers some of these same items that are used in the work. It is *all* conjuring. The root doctor usually took care of all the community's needs. They worked to cure and curse. It goes hand in hand.

Over the years I have slid some of the remedies my mama used to treat us with in a few of my books. I didn't go into great detail about or even explain why I added them or what they have to do with the work other than the basic information. It's all herbal, my dears! I'm gonna share some of the remedies here I grew up with and a little bit of information.

So here are the ingredients of Conjure: treating the community ills with remedies, the food and the way it is cooked, and the work. This all makes up Conjure—if you take one part out, then you've got half-baked cake! Some of these herbal ingredients that were used to heal could also be used in a trick to make the target ill. You have to understand that just because the ancestors were slaves together didn't mean they all got along. There was tricking going on inside those communities. The root doctor was honored and feared, but they were an important part of the community.

Many of the recipes the ancestors had to work with were dangerous. They had to be skilled in the treatment of others. They didn't have any written medical documentation like the white folks did. Their skills were something they were blessed with. I don't know where my mama learned how to treat us. I never asked her. I only remember going to the doctor once growing up and that was to the dentist to have a tooth pulled. My grandmas had a touch of healing in them to, and again I must say I'm not sure where the knowledge came from. Maybe it came from working in the fields or passed down in the family. All I know is that they treated us as children and kept us safe and well.

This work is so engrained into the culture that it is hard to separate. To be honest, growing up was a little hard sometimes 'cause folks thought my mama was weird. She had some funny ways, but I see myself with them, too. I didn't understand as a child, but I understand as an adult. My mama kept her culture alive and to some it made her look backwards and uneducated. She was standoffish and kept her business to herself, but there was a never-ending flow of folks coming and going from our home. We were not allowed to be in the house when strangers came calling; we had to be outside on the stoop. When folks came to see my mama, they always sat in the kitchen at the table.

The information below is old-school and should not be used without a skilled doctor. Some of these remedies can burn the skin or cause other adverse effects. Use common sense and wisdom when you are dealing with any kind of roots or herbs. If an illness appears, contact your local medical physician. I am in no way promoting self-treatment; this information is for learning purposes only. Before anyone has something smart to say about that, remember I am following the law of the land. I am *not* a medical doctor nor do I have a license to prescribe prescriptions.

There are a lot of old remedies that may seem silly in today's world, but in the old days it is what the ancestors had to work with. It is how they kept their families and others in the community healthy and well. You will see how Conjure flows over into everything dealing with the home—it truly is a way of life. I hope this information is useful.

I have to start with the one treatment I hated as a child and a grown-up. My mama dosed us every year with it, and sometimes within the year if we seemed to have a stomach ailment that just wouldn't go away. It is gross and leaves a lasting taste in your mouth. Although it is used for other things, this was one of the main uses.

Castor Oil

Jonah 4 V 6-7

6 And the Lord God prepared a gourd "castor bean tree", and made it to come up over Jonah, that it might be a shadow over his head, to deliver him from his grief. So Jonah was exceeding glad of the gourd.

7 But God prepared a worm when the morning rose the next day, and it smote the gourd that it withered.

Castor oil comes from the castor bean. When I was a child, it was given to us to make sure we were worm-free and our systems were cleaned out. Castor was also given for constipation and to moth-ers in labor that was not moving as it should. I was given it by my grandma when my labor wouldn't get harder; that is why women expecting children should never take castor oil.

The castor bean has a few different names: *Ricinus commu-nis*, the castor bean, Pammy Christy Bean, which comes from Palma Christi bean, or castor oil plant.

The old folks say the castor bean is lucky and holds magic.

Love Bag

You need a red bag. To the bag add a photo of your target, run a nail through the photo and say your petition, then add the photo to the bag. To this add three castor beans and some cotton that you have fed whiskey-soaked crossroads dirt.

Bury the bag under the roots of a rosebush for three days. On the fourth day as the sun is rising, dig up the bag. It is said that the roots of the rosebush and the rising sun will bring forth an undying love.

Lil Love Bundle

You can tie lavender, honeysuckle and rose petals along with the hair on the crown of your head into a small bundle with three knots to bring love. The cloth should be white. Place the bundle in your bosom near your heart.

Things to Make 'Em Swell

As most know, placing a brick in water can make a target swell. Did you know that yeast and peach tree leaves can do the same thing? This can be done by making a mud dollie.

Toothache Tree

The leaf from the "toothache tree" can be chewed to dull the ache of a toothache. The leaves from the toothache tree can also be worked with in all shut your mouth and stop gossip work.

Toothache

Cloves that have been soaked with a little whiskey can be placed in a small piece of white cloth and put on the affected tooth to relieve the pain. You have to be very careful with cloves because they can burn the skin. Never apply cloves to bare skin.

In conjure work cloves are added to works to heat them up. Don't get heavy-handed with them because they are very hot and could cause friction and trouble. Yet when cloves are added to a ham, they draw forth warmth and love within a family.

Orange Balls

I'm sure some of you remember the oranges covered in cloves around the holidays, commonly called pomanders. Did you now that those are conjure balls? Those are made for attraction and protection. They were mostly made for the holidays near the New Year. You make a small hole in an orange and place your petition in the hole. Then you cover the orange with cloves, and as you stick each clove into the orange, you say your prayers and petition. Then you hang the ball up and let it do its work.

Hard to Breathe

If we got a chest cold when we were young, my mama would treat us. She would put a plaster on your chest. You should never place them on your bare skin; mama always placed them on a white cloth. It seemed like everything had to be mixed with lard. For any issue dealing with a cough, congested chest, or just a cold so it wouldn't go to your chest, she would make a pine plaster. The plaster consisted of pine tips and lard; it really didn't smell too bad.

She would boil a little of the pine and steep it. Then she took a little of the water and mixed it with the lard and some of the pine tips. This was slathered on a white cloth, folded in half, and placed on our chest with the cover pulled up to our necks. And we would sweat. I'm not sure how long she left it on us. It seemed like forever, but I'm sure it wasn't.

She would also place pine tips in a pot of water in the wintertime and keep it on a low fire. The house always smelled so good. Pine sap can also be used to stop bleeding. My mama knew all those tricks, and she used the knowledge from her culture to keep us healthy.

Another treatment for breathing issues is "possum fat." Yep, you heard me. Possum fat helps with asthma and bronchitis. You need an old possum, and he needs to be killed after sundown but before midnight. Then you skin him and put him in a pot of hot water. Boil him until the meat is falling off the bones. Then you turn the fire off and let the water cool. As the water cools, the fat will make a film on top of the water just like a chicken does when you boil it. Once the fat has risen, you skim it out of the pot. Mix the grease with a pinch of sulfur and some ash from an oak limb. Mix the ingredients well while praying, and then you rub the grease on the back and chest covering it with a white sheet.

Mustard Seed Plaster

A mustard seed plaster is used to draw. You soak the seed in a little water with a drop or two of olive oil added to it. Pray Mark 4 V 30-32 over the bowl. Let the seeds sit for about an hour, then drain them and mash the seeds into a paste. You then spread the paste on a white cloth and place the cloth on the affected area. A mustard seed plaster can be used to draw out colds also. Be very careful because it will blister the skin and should only be left on for no longer than five minutes at a time.

> *30 And He said, "How shall we picture the kingdom of God, or by what parable shall we present it?"*
>
> *31 "It is like a mustard seed, which, when sown upon the soil, though it is smaller than all the seeds that are upon the soil,*
>
> *32 yet when it is sown, it grows up and becomes larger than all the garden plants and forms large branches; so that the birds of the air can nest under the shade."*

Sassafras

I love this stuff! I love the smell and the power of it. It can heal or kill. Up until the mid-1970s you could buy it at the drugstores in the rural South, and then they stopped selling it. You may be asking: how can it kill? When I was in school in South Carolina back in the day, head lice was bad. It was out of control. There wasn't any of the treatments they have today. My hair was down to my waist and curly. I got them at school, and my grandma gave me two options: either cut my hair or get it treated.

I was not gonna cut my hair; so my sister got a ride and went to town to the drugstore to get some more sassafras oil because grandma only had one bottle and that wasn't enough for my hair. My grandma covered my head in the oil and then wrapped my head in a white towel. She left the treatment on my hair for about three hours, then we washed my hair. There were tons of them in the washtub. I have never had them again. That is the only thing other than tea tree oil I know of that kills the eggs, too.

Sassafras tea settles the stomach and some stay it will keep your body running right. It can also be added to soups and gumbo to give them a wonderful flavor.

Mud Plaster

Did you know that mud mixed with sweetgrass will draw out infection in boils and infected areas? It is also good for swelling. River or creek mud is the best. Gather your mud and sweetgrass, get a lil jar of river water so you can add it to the mud if it starts to dry. Using your hands and praying as you work that the swelling or infection be pulled out, mix the mud and sweetgrass together.

Once it is mixed well, put some on a white cloth, and place the cloth on the affected area. Don't let the plaster touch the skin. Leave the cloth on the affected area until the mud dries; then remove the cloth. The patient will be able to feel the pull as the plaster does its job.

Another way to pull out infection is to place a piece of fatback in between a white cloth and then tape it to the affected area for twenty-four hours. Let the area breathe and repeat the process with a new wrap until the infection is drawn out.

Remedies That Draw

The sap from a sweet gum tree mixed with lard can be applied using a white cloth to help with inflammation; it also helps with sores and cuts that are getting infected. Do not apply directly to the skin.

Tobacco is another herb that works wonderful to draw out poisons from small insect bites or boils. Have the person spit on the tobacco, then place it over the area that needs to be treated. Then take the white of an egg and place it on a white cloth. Wrap the cloth around the area. The cloth simply holds the egg white in place until it dries.

Tar and lard mixed together can be used to draw out infections in the skin. The tar pulls out the infection; it should never be applied directly on the skin because it will burn the skin. Always place it on a white cloth so the cloth is in contact with the skin.

Bundle for Peace

I leave this section with a recipe for a bundle of peace to hang in your home. To a white handkerchief add dirt from your land, bay leaf, a dove feather, and some hair from the crown of your head. Gather the four corners and pull them tightly together; then use red cotton string to wrap around the top of the bundle to close it. Tie the knots in the name of the Holy Trinity. Then feed the bundle either coffee or a little whiskey. You can place it anywhere in your home, but hanging it from the bedpost is traditional.

Headache Tree

When I was growing up, I suffered with bad headaches—what I now know as migraines. Back in that time there was no money to go to the doctor, and most folks didn't trust them. My mama treated me with leaves of the headache tree. She would cut two leaves from the tree, then I had to spit on each leaf one at the time and place them on my temples.

I would have to lay down with the room dark and a white cloth with sweet oil on it placed across my forehead. I remember no matter how hard I tried to stay awake, I always fell asleep. When I would wake up, my head felt so much better.

Cut N Remove Sprinkle/Wash/Spray

Heat a pot of water on the stove, then bring it to a boil. When the water starts to boil, turn the fire off. Add four tablespoons of cream of tartar and four tablespoons of soda. Stir the water going in the backwards direction, then cover the pot. Once the water has cooled, squeeze the lemon into the mix. Stir the mixture well, then pour it into mop water or a spray bottle and clean your home. Remember to dress all your windows and doors after this strong cleansing. You can also sprinkle this around your home and yard to cut and clear anything that might be there.

Cut N Clear Powder

You need the dirt from the four corners of the crossroads, soda ash, your petition burnt to ash, and cream of tartar. Mix all the ingredients together and sprinkle the powder in the four directions leading away from your home to cut and clear a jinx or crossed condition.

To Cure Pink Eye

Breast milk dropped in the eye three times a day will cure pink eye. It will also sooth the burning and irritation in the eye.

To Cure a Sty

Clean your ear and rub the wax over the infected sty. Do this for five days.

To See If You Have Conceived

Hold a needle over your stomach, and thread the needle with red thread over the stomach area while praying. Then hold the pendulum over the stomach; if the pendulum moves, then you need to get checked out and start vitamins.

Christ in the Cradle

Wrap a leaf from the Christ in the cradle plant around your petition. Be very careful 'cause the plant can make you itch. Place the wrapped petition on a small white cloth and add the rest of the ingredients. This work can be done for anything you need help with.

Teething Baby

THIS IS FOR INFORMATION USE ONLY

Braid three equal pieces of red cotton string together. On each braid pray the Trinity and petition for the baby (who you call by name) to cut their teeth without pain. You need a large button with four holes in it. Run the strings through one hole to the other on each side. Then tie the string around the baby's neck.

Chicken Fat Rub

I call this rub the cure-all rub. I don't know how it works, but it does. It works on all kind of ailments from constipation to muscular pain and everything in between. This is always kept in my cabinet. My family doesn't really care for it because it smells kind of bad; but I use it when the need arises.

It is made from a farm-fresh boiled chicken. A store-bought chicken will not work. You boil the chicken until it is done, then turn the fire off and let the chicken sit until the water has become cold and the fat from the chicken has risen to the top of the pot. Then you skim the fat off the top of the water and place it in a jar. You can have chicken salad for dinner with the chicken.

Add three tablespoons of olive oil to the chicken fat while call-ing on the Trinity with each spoon added: the first spoon for God the Father, the second spoon for God the Son, the third spoon for God the Holy Spirit or Holy Ghost. Then you add three bay leaves and repeat the process as you did with the olive oil. In the old days when I was first taught this, I was taught to set it outside in the sun for twenty-one days. Then you remove the bay leaves, and it is ready to use.

However, with today's fast-paced world, I now place the jar in a double boiler and heat the oil on a low flame for about five hours. Sometimes I leave the bay leaves in the jar, and sometimes I take them out. It all depends. When you rub the oil on the area where there is pain, you will find that the smell tends to not matter at all because the oil feels warm and soothing, and before you know it, the pain is gone.

Breathe with Ease

You can burn the Fussy Gussy leaves over charcoal to help with colds, sore throats, and other ailments of the chest. You can also add it to a pot of water and boil it on the stove to open up stopped-up sinuses. It can also be added to a pillow to help you breathe easy at night. Fussy Gussy is just an old country name for life everlasting.

A Conjure Worker's First-Aid Kit

BAKING SODA: used for baths, washes, and powders; employed in drawing works and uncrossing works.

BIBLE: The ancestors hid the work within the pages of the Old Testament. The work is not built on the Bible; the work is hidden in the Bible. The Bible is a large part of Conjure.

BONES: raccoon bones, possum, chicken, gator, cat, dog, and many other bones.

BORAX: Twenty Mule Team Borax can be added to all types of works for added power and in works to remove.

BROOM: a must for all cleansing and protection.

CANDLES: white, red, blue, orange, green, black, purple, and tealights.

CORNSTARCH: can be worked with for all types of cleansing works and can be a base for making powders.

CREAM OF TARTAR: worked with for all removing works and can be worked with for crossing.

DIRTS: bank, courthouse, crossroads, stop sign, church.

HERBS: Master of the Woods, Solomon's seal, calamus, frankincense and myrrh, five finger grass, lovage, orange peel, lemongrass, alum, damiana, lavender, dried red pepper, devil's bit, devil's shoestring, High John, Low John, Dixie John, patchouli, rue, rosemary, cinnamon, and angelica root.

MARKER: to mark the spot and the target.

NAILS: to nail down the work and the targets. Also used in conjure waters.

NEEDLE: are worked with as a pendulum or to nail something down.

OILS: protection, love, money, domination, run devil run, reversal, success.

PAPER: for petitions

PENCIL WITH NO ERASER: I was taught to always write a petition with a pencil that had no eraser so the work couldn't be erased.

PLAYING CARDS: You need a deck of playing cards so you can hear the ancestors speak.

RED COTTON STRING: used to tie, bind, and wrap.

RED FLANNEL: to make packets, bags, mojo bags, and dollies.

SALT: can draw blessings or can cross.

SCISSORS: used to cut and clear things out of the way and for protection.

SODA ASH: worked with for all types of cleansing work.

VINEGAR: can be worked with for cleansing or crossing.

WATERS: holy, storm, stagnant, sweet, blue.

WHITE HANDKERCHIEF: for making packets and praising the spirits.

WOODS: weeping willow, witch hazel, oak, pine, lightning struck, pecan.

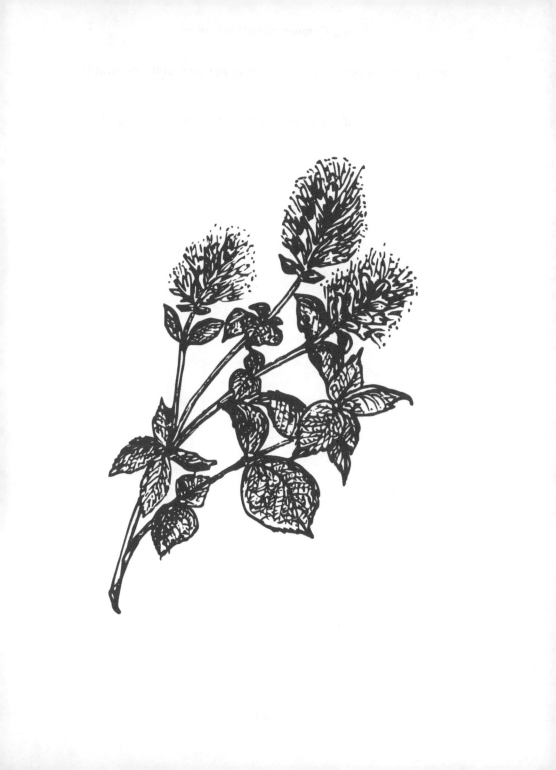

CURIOS, TOOLS, AND MISCELLANEOUS INGREDIENTS

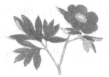

ALLIGATOR CLAW: An alligator claw is carried for drawing good luck and money workings. It is said by the old folks that an alligator claw can pick up good luck. So this claw is a good one to carry for all prosperity work.

ALLIGATOR TOOTH: A necklace made with an alligator tooth is said to be very lucky. The old folks say that it will draw good luck in every aspect of the wearer's life. Sometimes this is even added to conjure packets, especially in gambling hands.

ALUM POWDER: Alum stops gossip and stops folks from talking out of the sides of their mouth at you. Alum is very bitter and worked with for all backstabbing work. It is also worked to bust loose from crossed conditions that can't seem to be removed. This is one of my favorite to work with in shut your mouth work.

AMMONIA: Ammonia is a powerful cleanser! It can be employed for general cleansing for altars, homes, and businesses. It is used to remove crossed conditions, jinxes, and all forms of evil. Ammonia is one of those cleansers that bust away all blocks and crossed conditions.

ANIMAL PARTS: Animal bones have been worked with in Conjure since the beginning whether they are being worked for drawing luck or for adding spiritual power to the Work. They are added to all types of work from conjure bags to medicine bottles. Here are a few examples: chicken feet are worked with for cleansing, an alligator's claw is for luck and to draw in money works, the rabbit's foot is always lucky, and chicken eggs are worked with to help pull things away from the client in spiritual cleansing work.

BADGER TEETH: Badger teeth are good for gambler's luck.

BITTERS: Understanding bitter ingredients—both plants and other things—is very important. I have seen some confusion about adding bitter herbs to love works and other works. If an herb or a root is bitter, then that herb or root should only be worked with on souring or cleansing works. If something is bitter, then it is going to leave a bitter taste in your mouth, so to say. So why in the world would you add something of this type to a work where you are trying to draw a loved one in or for prosperity and success works? I'm sorry but it just does not make sense to me. I was taught that bitter herbs and roots are worked with in all types of cleansing, reversals, and enemy works; I was not taught to work with them for positive works. Bitter ingredients you can look up individually in this book are alum, ammonia, black coffee, lemon, Lysol, Murphy's Oil Soap, Mrs. Stewart's Bluing, Pine-Sol, red devil lye, tar water, and vinegar.

BONES: Animal parts have been a great source for drawing luck and adding spiritual power to conjure work and conjure bags. And bones make up a big part of this. Bones are powerful. Bones have been worked with to find out what is going on since the throwing of lots in the Bible. You can find references to this in 1 Samuel 14 V 40–42, Proverbs 16 V 33, Proverbs 18 V 18, and Acts 1 V 26, just to name a few. We work with bones to tell the future and also for help within our conjure work. Bones are thrown in Conjure to find out what ails the client; in a way, this is a type of divination. As a young worker, I was taught to read the bones, and later on in years I started working with them as a full-blown divination tool. The bones are a way for our ancestors to communicate with us. You have to remember that the bone from an animal still holds the spirit of that animal.

Working with animal bones can help him power your conjure work. There is much to be learned from animals and their habits and how these can be applied in Conjure. When you add these bones to your work, you are adding the spirit of that animal to your work.

- BLACK CAT BONE: Black cat bones are a prize among all Conjures; this is a valuable bone. The black cat bone is one of my favorite bones to work with; it is alleged to bring luck, power, success, and money. For me it is one of my lucky bones. In the old days it was said that the carcass had to be thrown in a pot of boiling water. Then the first bone that floated to the surface was a powerful bone and was to be carried for good luck. I was taught a little different. I was taught that all black cat bones are powerful. They can be carried for everything from luck to protection. These are something to be cherished and taken very good care of. The longer you have them, the stronger their work with you will be.

- CHICKEN BONES: Some conjure workers work with the chicken bones in bone reading. I was taught to work with them for protection. You can make a protection cross to place behind your door that will keep enemies away from your door. You need two thigh bones and some red cotton thread. Place the bones in a red ant bed and let the ants remove all the flesh from the bones. Then bring the bones in and cleanse them under some cool running water.

  The next step in this work is to set the bones on your ancestor altar for three days. The first day you put the bones side by side. The second day you put the bones in the shape of a cross. Place them one on top of the other, which will make the four arms of the cross. On the third day you will take your red thread and wrap it around the center of the bones. The best way that I have found to do this is to wrap three times one way and then cross over and wrap the other way three times. You just repeat the process until the bones are held secure by the red cotton thread. Tie three knots in your cotton thread.

  Place your cross in a tealight setup with five tealights. Four of the tealights are placed one each at the end of each arm of your cross, and one is placed on top of the cross where the red thread holds the cross together. Leave the cross on your ancestor altar for another twenty-four hours. Feed your cross with some whiskey, and then you can take it and nail the cross either behind your front door or above it. Once a month take down the cross and repeat the instructions. Leave the cross on your ancestor altar for three days so they can feed it and empower it, then put it back where you had it.

- CHICKEN FEET: Chicken feet are worked with in all types of conjure work. They can draw, or they can remove. The thing that you really need to remember is that the chicken is constantly scratching; they scratch and peck all day long. That's how they spend their days. They are very good when you are doing a spiritual cleansing. All you have to do is scratch yourself lightly moving downward from the crown of your head to the bottom of your feet with a chicken foot. This will scratch off anything that has been sent your way by an enemy. Chicken feet are a good way to keep your daily cleansings up without having to take long drawn-out baths. They are also hung in cars to keep the driver safe and all crossed conditions away from the car.

- COON BONES: Raccoon bones are worked with in Conjure as a tool for divination. There are some old workers who prefer coon bones in bone throwing instead of possum bones. I guess the one thing that coon bones are well-known for—thanks to the internet—is the penis bone. It is said that this bone is very powerful in all types of love works or gambling hands. I have one in my set of possum bones that I perform bone readings with. I have found that the penis bone represents different types of situations within a reading depending on how it falls.

- HORNS: Horns make wonderful containers. They can be worked with for everything from protection work to love work. They work well because they are hard to destroy.

Once you have the work done and placed inside the horn, you can hang the horn up anywhere in your home. This type of work is good when you are trying to get the target next to the work without them realizing that they are being worked on. That's what is called a trick. Conjure workers are famous for being tricky.

- POSSUM BONES: Possom bones are a divination tool in Conjure. I was taught to read bones with either coon bones or possum bones. I think out of them both I prefer possum bones. They seem to show when something is being hidden within a reading. Possum bones are also worked with when you are trying to hide something. If you are doing a job and you need to be able to be unnoticed, then you would work with a possum bone because everyone knows that the possum is very good at being ignored. Most of the time we think they are dead when really all they are doing is acting dead.

- RABBIT'S FOOT: Everyone knows about the rabbit's foot and the tale of how lucky it is. I think of all the curios in Conjure the rabbit's foot is the most famous. A rabbit's foot is said to bring success and happiness but also protection from one's enemies. The rabbit foot can be placed behind your door of your home to draw forth all things needed within that home. You can take a five-dollar bill and wrap it around a foot with the face looking outward. Use red cotton string to secure the bill to the foot. Then feed the foot some whiskey and hang it behind your front door. Speak to the face on the dollar bill and tell them to go and find you some money. Refresh the work once a month by taking it down and feeding it some whiskey; then hang it back up.

BROOMS: This spiritual cleansing tool sweeps away unwanted spirits and enemies. It is good for an all-around protection of the home. A broom can be placed behind the door with the head up to keep folks away.

CHALK: Chalk is used to mark items in your work and on your altar for blessing or crossing. It is also used to mark windows and doors for protection.

CHAMBER LYE: Some workers like to use their urine in works. My issue is that urine sours. So what happens when the urine in the work goes bad?

CHAMPAGNE: Champagne is given as an offering as payment for a successful job.

CLAY: Clay is worked with in making dollies and also to nail a target down.

COFFEE, BLACK: is one of my favorite blockbusting washes. Black coffee is well-known to strip away and bust open all blocks that could possibly be holding you back. This is one of the strongest ingredients in any wash that I know of that not only cleanses but also removes jinxes and blocks.

COINS: Pennies and dimes are used as payment or offerings to ancestors and crossroads spirits. The quarter is a powerful coin as it can be multiplied by the number five. The number five is very important as it represents the crossroads and the spirit that lives there: the four corners plus the spirit in the center equals five.

CONJURE BAG: Conjure bags—also called hands—are made for a variety of conditions. A red flannel or leather packet is put together and loaded with roots, herbs, dirts, and other fixed items based on what you are looking for. These can be worn for protection, healing, love, or luck.

CONJURE STICK: In old-style Conjure this is used when working with Moses or petitioning other biblical prophets; brings power and control to your work. It is used to call down the spirit into your work.

DOLLIES: The dollie is as old as time. Dollies can be made for healing, luck, love, enemy work, protection, and a variety of other conjure needs. They are made to represent an individual to target blessings or curses to. The spirit of the target is pulled down into the dollie. Dollies come in all shapes and sizes, and they can be made out of whatever material you have on hand such as wax, cloth, clay, mud, and even dried apples.

DIRT DAUBER NEST: is worked with in all domination work, but it is also good in enemy work. It adds extra power to all work.

DIRT: Dirts are worked with in all types of work from hotfoot work to healing work. It is mixed with powders, herbs, and sprinkled where a target will get into it. In the old days dirt was collected from many different places. Dirts are a large part of Conjure, although it seems New Age workers don't deal with them as much as the workers from days gone by. It seems that the only dirts most folk work with now are either graveyard dirt or those dealing with the law. There are many more dirts out there to be worked with for a variety of conditions. If you are interested in this work and you want to make the products the old way, then you are gonna have to go out and collect what you need.

- BANK DIRT: This is good for all money works; anything you need money to buy or pay. It can help with financial security and can also be worked with to cross up someone's cash.

- CHURCH DIRT: Church dirt is worked with for all your spiritual needs, even love work and money works. Used for blessings, healings, and protection work, it can help in repairing broken relationships as well.

- COURTHOUSE DIRT: All justice and court case work benefits from courthouse dirt. It can also be worked with to stir up trouble for a target.

- CROSSROADS DIRT: This can open or close a target's road. It can also be worked with to stop a target.

- DIRT FROM FIGHTING DOGS' YARD: This dirt is worked with to cause the target confusion and to cause fighting and destruction.

- FIRE ANT DIRT: Dirt from a fire ant mound is worked with to draw or remove something or to stir things up and heat them up.

- GRAVEYARD DIRT: Graveyard dirt is worked with for a variety of reasons—both for the right hand and the left.

- HOSPITAL DIRT: Hospital dirt is worked with for all healing work but can be worked with for darker justified works too.

- POLICE STATION DIRT: All justice work can use police station dirt. This dirt can be worked with to either bring the law or in law stay away work.

- RAILROAD TRACK DIRT: This dirt can be worked with to draw or send away.

- RIVER DIRT: River dirt can be worked for cleansing, making a dollie, or bogging a target down.

- SNAKE DIRT: If you are lucky enough to find a snake crossing, scoop up as much dirt as possible. You can work with this dirt for wisdom, protection, knowledge, and enemy works.

- TERMITE DIRT: Termite dirt is good to tear down an enemy's foundation, to strip away their personal power.

EGGS: Eggs can be used to cleanse or to cross someone up. Wiping yourself down with an egg and then throwing the egg in the crossroads will cleanse and remove crossed conditions. They are worked with in healing, curse removal, jinx-removing, uncrossing work, and crossing work.

FIRE ANTS: Fire ants, also called piss ants, can be worked with to drive someone away, draw in blessings, and get the target moving. They are used for carrying messages and petitions or running someone out of your life. Fire ants will work hard to carry your petition where it needs to go. They are also good for heating things up.

FLOOR SWEEPS: Floor sweeps are an important tool in workings. You don't hear much about floor sweeps in the work anymore, but they are a powerhouse to work with. So much is being lost in this tradition. Sweeps can be worked with as an easy way to either draw something into the home or sweep it out.

GUNPOWDER: Gunpowder—used carefully—will get things moving. It also heats up a work and will provide quick activation—an explosion of power. It can be used in all blockbuster work. Gunpowder is very dangerous to use: it is placed here for information purposes only.

HOLY OIL: This blessed oil is used for dressing the sick and for protection and candle dressing as well. Usually olive oil is the base.

JARS AND POTS: A variety of these are used for all container work.

LIGHTNING STRUCK WOOD: Any lightning struck wood adds extra power to a work, but oak gives extra power and strength.

LODESTONE: These stones made of magnetic iron ore are used for drawing and attracting in Conjure although they have a weaker pull than a magnet. They can be added to all works to draw love, money, and luck.

LYSOL (ORIGINAL BROWN): My children literally hate the smell of brown Lysol. It is one of the staples in my conjure cabinet. My oldest son is forty-three years old, and he still remembers the smell of Lysol all through the house when he was a child. Like ammonia this is one of the strongest spiritual cleansers you're going to find. You don't see many talking about it today. It is about forgotten. Like coffee and ammonia, Lysol will bust open those blocks, and it also offers protection. This is a cleanser that should be used once a week at least in your home or business. It is used in sprays and washes to spiritual cleanse and wash away crossed conditions.

MAGNET: Magnets have a stronger pull than a lodestone—because of that stronger pull they will draw faster. They are worked with to draw prosperity, money, love, or anything else the worker may need.

MIRRORS: Mirrors are worked with for protection works and for all types of binding work. They are helpful for reversal works.

MRS. STEWART'S BLUING: For uses in protection, cleansings, and luck. A few drops of bluing can be placed in a jar of water, then put on your reading table to help draw Spirit.

MURPHY'S OIL SOAP: Murphy's Oil Soap is used for spiritual cleansing of a home and business and also helps with cutting and clearing. Murphy's contains lemongrass, so it is good for all-around cleansings. It is also good on all woodwork, so it is safe to use to wash down walls and floors.

NAILS: Nails are worked with to pin folks down. Rusty nails can be used in bottle conjure to cross someone up. The old square-headed nails can be made into a cross by binding them together with red cotton string to then hang at front and back doors for protection.

OIL LAMP: One of the oldest tools used in Conjure, oil lamps can be burned for love, money, protection, domination, or any other condition or situation where a steady flame is needed. Herbs, roots, and other items can be added to the oil lamp base for specific workings. Like candle burning, there are a variety of works that can be done using an oil lamp. One of the best things about the lamp is that you can keep a steady low flame going on the work.

PINE-SOL (ORIGINAL): This is good for all types of spiritual cleansings, money drawing, and uncrossing work. It will leave your home or business feeling refreshed, and it has a nice clean smell to it.

PERSONAL CONCERNS: Personal concerns are any items you have that give you a direct connection to your target. That includes blood, sexual fluids, photos, hair, used garments, chamber lye, spit, and their foot tracks.

PINS AND NEEDLES: These tools are worked with to nail a target down or to get your point across. They are worked with in all types of things from dollie work to crossing work. They can even be used as a pendulum.

POWDERS: Powders are worked with for hotfoot workings, sachet powders, and floor sweeps. Powders are made by mixing dirts, roots, and herbs together in a base powder.

PYRITE: Pyrite is helpful for drawing good fortune, money, and success in business.

RAILROAD SPIKES: Railroad spikes are forged of hot iron. That makes them unbendable They are worked with in many types of conjure work—both with the left hand and the right. They are very powerful for all types of protection but also can be worked with to draw or to send away. They nail things down and can be employed for crossing work.

RED BRICK DUST: Red brick dust is used for protection. Mixed with dirts and herbs, red brick dust can be sprinkled across doorways and around the yard for blessing and keeping enemies out.

RED DEVIL LYE: Red devil lye is used for protection work concerning the home and property. It is also good for getting rid of bill collectors, enemies, and all things unwanted. It's hard to find nowadays, but you can get it at some of the feed stores. In the old days this product was buried at the four corners of a house or the four corners of a property with the devil on the label always facing outward. The old folks say that at the sight of it the devil himself would be sent running. The red devil on the front of those lye bottles has become the imagery for the run devil run products worked with today in conjure work.

RED FLANNEL: Red flannel is what is traditionally used to make dollies, packets, and conjure bags.

SALT: This is the biblical powerhouse of spiritual blessing and cleansing. The use of salt guarantees our blessings, preservation, and protection under God. Salt can also jinx. Don't forget what happen to Lot's wife.

SALTPETER: Saltpeter is used in uncrossing works and to tie a man's nature.

SCISSORS: Scissors are used to cut away illness and crossed conditions. They can also provide protection. Keep an opened pair on the front doorframe of your house and they will cut any crossed conditions sent your way as well as cutting away malice from folks entering your home or business.

SKELETON KEY: These keys are used for a variety of conjure working. An iron skeleton key can be used as a pendulum for opening all doors to insights. Keys bound in red cotton string can be placed either above or beside the door to keep all roads open. Use them in conjure workings with Saint Peter, who opens all doors and roadways.

STRING: String is very useful for tying down or for cutting and clearing crossed conditions. It can also be worked with to clear the roads by cutting one piece away at a time. In old-style Conjure, red, black, and white are the colors for string used in a variety of works.

SULFUR: Sulfur is used for removing unwanted spirits from a place, all enemy work, hotfoot powders as well as crossing conjure. It can also be placed in the corners of a room for protection. Sulfur is worked with when you need to clear an area that has been crossed or has unruly spirits that won't leave. A pinch of sulfur behind the door will help protect the home from cross conditions and false friends.

SWEETENERS: Syrups, sugars, and honey are used in all types of sweetening work. Some particular sweeteners from the plant world are:

- APPLE: Sweetens and used in love workings or works of power.

- HONEYCOMB: Used in sweetening work as well as domination workings, to get the upper hand; can be worked with as a trap. A honeycomb can be wrapped around the photo of a target you want to sweeten and control.

- ORANGES: Good for all attraction work.

- PEACHES: All sweetening work. The peach seed can also be worked with to cross up an enemy or separate a couple.

- POMEGRANATE: For love drawing, passion, and sexual attraction in conjure works.

- WATERMELON: Good for all sweetening work. The seed can be worked with to make a work grow.

VINEGAR: Used for protection from illness and as a spiritual cleanser. It is also worked with to sour a person, place, or situation. It is said that four-thieves vinegar will clear away all crossed conditions and spiritual illnesses.

WHISKEY: Whiskey is used in petitioning offerings to the ancestors and spirits. It is also worked with to feed conjure bags, dollies, and other ongoing works. Fireball Whiskey is good for all run devil run works and also to heat a work up. It can also be worked with to feed all money works.

WATERS: Waters are worked with for cleansings, washes, baths, blessings, and feeding the spirits. Herbs, coloring, and perfumes can also be added to the water. Bluing is a good example: it is worked with in a reading to draw Spirit closer.

- BLUE WATER: Blue water is used to see the spirit and also for protection.

- DISHWATER: Dishwater thrown out the front door of the home stops fighting inside the home. If there is fussing and fighting in the home, then after supper wash the dishes in a dishpan and throw the water out the front door. It can also be worked with for cleansing and releasing work.

- DITCH WATER/STAGNANT WATER: These waters are worked with to keep an enemy down, to stop them. They are also worked with for bindings, confusion, crossing, and general enemy work.

- FRESH WATERS: Well water, spring water, rainwater, and creek water are all used to refresh the spirit of one's work and to draw things needed.

- HOLY WATER: Blessed water is good for protection, healings, and adding power to your conjure work.

- HURRICANE WATER: Just like a hurricane, this type of water can be worked with to stir up an enemy's life or to turn their world upside down.

- LIGHTNING WATER: Lightning water is worked with in the same way storm water is, to stir up messes and to start fussing and fighting. It can also be worked with to battle your way out of a situation. Be careful because you might heat up the work too much.

- RIVER WATER: River water will refresh the spirit for cleansing works. It is also worked with to remove things or to send a target away.

- STORM WATER: is worked with to stir up messes and to start fussing and fighting. It can also be worked with to battle your way out of a situation.

- STUMP WATER: Like ditch water, this is one of those double-hands ingredients: you can work with it for a variety of works from crossings to healing.

- TAR WATER: Tar water is for sticking an enemy where they can't move forward and also for protection and uncrossing. You can also work with it for all crossing works, blocks, and jinx work. Tar water is like a double-edged sword: it can be worked with for good or for harder works depending on the situation. You can add it to your mop water and cleanse your home from back to front to remove all crossed conditions. You can pour some tar water in a mason jar and set the uncapped jar behind your front door; this will strip away the power of any enemy that comes through that front door.

- TOILET WATER: Good for all types of work; it just depends on what you are doing.

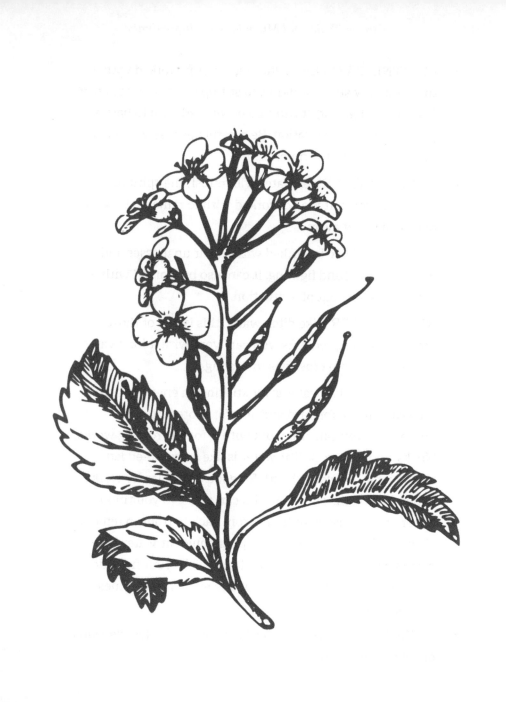

PRAYERS
AND PETITIONS

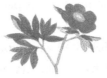

Prayers and petitions are at the center of conjure work. Prayers are the biblical verses you recite to power up ingredients and work as well as some other litanies of the church. Petitions are your own requests in your own words for what you need. How you write or say your petition is important. I've gone into that in my other books. In short, always make sure your petition is clear and to the point. Be careful of what you are asking for, and make yourself very clear on what it is you want to bring into your life. You have to remember that Spirit will bring you exactly what you ask for, so you don't want there to be any confusion.

In this section, I will share with you some prayers I want you to know as well as some works that go along with the biblical figures I have worked with.

Moses: God's Two-Headed Worker

Since the days of slavery, old conjure workers and poor folk alike have regarded Moses as one of the most powerful conjure workers ever born because Moses spoke directly to God and he allowed God to use him to help his people. He was even allowed to see God's back. Moses obtained many gifts through which miracles took place. God used Moses to restore the faith of his people and lead them to the Promised Land.

Moses, like all God's folk, had a mission assigned to him by God. Moses was sent by God to deliver his people and set them free. Moses had a throw-down with pharaoh's magicians because they challenged God's authority. He worked his conjure stick to hammer pharaoh and his army. By Moses calling on God, that conjure stick turned into snakes. This tells us that Moses can defeat any enemy known and unknown.

Moses can be petitioned for any situation where you need a helping hand. If you feel defeated or left out in the desert—or maybe you feel deserted—Moses is the one to petition and call for help. He will lead you out of despair into the land of milk and honey.

This work comes from the Old Testament. I want to share some that I haven't seen written about, nor do I think most folks even know about it. This is the marking of windows and doors. My mama always wiped our doors and washed the walls and such in our home a couple of times a year. The marking of the doors comes from Exodus 12 V 1-14 and the Passover and the Festival of Unleavened Bread. In Exodus 12 V 1-13 Moses was given instructions for this. There are a couple of important things the people were instructed to do. In verse 2 we see that God told Moses that this month would be the very first month in his year.

This month is to be for you the first month, the
first month of your year.

Then he goes on to give Moses instructions on what is to be done and when it is to be done. In verse 3 he orders a lamb for each family; then in verse 4 he says if the family is small, they should share with another family.

3 Tell the whole community of Israel that on the
tenth day of this month each man is to take a
lamb for his family, one for each household.

4 If any household is too small for a whole lamb,
they must share one with their nearest neighbor,
having taken into account the number of people
there are.

You are to determine the amount of lamb needed in accordance with what each person will eat.

In verses 5-6 he gives instructions on the type of animals that should be taken—either a goat or a sheep—and that they shouldn't be more than a year old. He also gives the day and time when they should be slaughtered. Twilight is when the sun has gone down; as a young worker I was taught that this is the time for removing.

5 The animals you choose must be year-old males
without defect. And you may take them from
sheep or the goats.

> *6 Take care of them until the fourteenth day of
> the month, when all the members of the commu-
> nity of Israel must slaughter them at twilight.*

In verse 7 Moses is given instructions for the doors to be marked with the blood from the animals. Some old folks when they mark their doors with chalk or oil will say on each mark, "I mark this door with the blood of the lamb," and as you will see further down in this writing, that is done for protection.

> *Then they are to take some of the blood and put
> it on the sides and tops of the doorframes of the
> houses where they eat the lambs.*

In verses 8–10 Moses is also instructed on how the food should be cooked. The meat shouldn't be eaten raw or boiled. It had to be roasted with bitter herbs. In conjure work bitter herbs are worked with for cleansing or for souring. I think here it is for cleansings. Nothing should be left over.

> *8 That same night they are to eat the meat
> roasted over the fire, along with bitter herbs, and
> bread made without yeast.*
>
> *9 Do not eat the meat raw or boiled in water, but
> roast it over a fire with the head, legs, and inter-
> nal organs.*
>
> *10 Do not leave any of it till morning; if some is
> left till morning, you must burn it.*

In verses 11–12 Moses is instructed on what he should wear while eating. This is where an understanding of the Bible is needed. This is also something that conjure workers are taught because the Old

Testament is where a lot of the work comes from. He is instructed to have his cloak "tucked" into his belt. If we tuck our cloak, then we are doing so for protection from the elements. He was also instructed to have his sandals on his feet. Our shoes protect us too. Then he was told to hold his staff in his hand while he ate. Everyone knows that Moses's staff was a magical rod which was worked for protection or destruction. He was also told to eat in a hurry 'cause the Lord was fixing to make a pass over the whole town. That is where the name of the Passover came from in the Bible. Moses is also told that those who do not have blood on their doors will be unprotected and their firstborn and their livestock firstborn will be struck down.

> 11 *This is how you are to eat it: with your cloak tucked into your belt, your sandals on your feet and your staff in your hand. Eat it in haste; it is the Lord's Passover.*
>
> 12 *"On that same night I will pass through Egypt and strike down every firstborn of both people and animals, and I will bring judgment on all the gods of Egypt. I am the Lord.*

In verse 13 God told Moses that anyone who had their doors marked would be protected and he would pass over those homes.

> *The blood will be a sign for you on the houses where you are, and when I see the blood, I will pass over you. No destructive plague will touch you when I strike Egypt.*

I wanted to offer a work in this section to honor Moses and my elders. You can use chalk or oil to dress your doors with. If you look in verse 7, you will see God told Moses exactly where the people should mark their doors. This is the same way I saw my mama, aunties, and my elders mark doors and windows:

> *Then they are to take some of the blood and put*
> *it on the sides and tops of the door frames of the*
> *houses where they eat the lambs.*

Make a wash with three bay leaves, four pinches of salt, and one olive leaf. Once the wash is cool, remove the herbs and set them to the side. Call on the Trinity, your ancestors, and Moses and petition them to clear away any conditions that are there with the wash. Petition them to remove anything that is not in accord with the spirits of the home. Use a white cloth to wipe down the front and back doors with the wash. Make sure you clean the inside and outside of each door. Remember to wipe in a downward motion. Start at the top of the door and pull downward and outward; do the same thing with the frames.

Once you have the doors and doorframes washed, you need to come back and close them. Sometimes, depending on what is going on, I may dress the doors with oil or a spray and then come back and mark them with my chalk. Do what you feel drawn to do. This is just a guide, not law!

I make crosses on my doors and windows with chalk or oil. Starting at the top of the doorframe draw the downward arm of the cross while calling on the Trinity, your ancestors, and Moses; petition them to protect your home and to destroy your enemies. Make the sideways arm of the cross while praying the same petition. I like to mark my doors top to bottom, the left to right because I want to lock down the doorway into my home. I mark the doorframes first, then I will come back and mark my doors.

This work is an easy way to keep your home well-protected and to have Moses stand guard at its entrances.

Moses in the Basket

You can also offer Moses a basket plant. Then you can feed the plant with your petitions and needs. The old folks say anything Moses could do, the plant can do. You write your petition out and petition Moses. Then you burn your petition to ash and place the ash in the soil of the plant. Give Moses an offering of a light, and as the plant grows, the work will become stronger.

The Blood of Jesus

There is nothing stronger than praying the blood of Jesus over someone. There is power in the blood that he shed for us upon the cross. No devil or demon can stand when covered with the precious blood of Jesus. I was taught at a very young age to plead the blood of Jesus on illnesses, nightmares, haunts, and anything else that I felt threatened by. Nothing can withstand being covered with the precious blood of Jesus. The Sacred Heart of Jesus is one of the strongest candles you can burn for enemy work and for healing. Even folks who are not Christian know that Jesus was very gifted. He was given the power to defeat death and bring forth life. He could feed a multitude with a piece of fish and a loaf of bread. So why in the world would folks think that his blood couldn't cure any illness or defeat any demon, devil, or enemy?

Below you will find a couple of prayers that I have worked with. You will be surprised at the power the blood of Jesus holds. There are a lot of folks who fear being covered with the blood of Jesus. These prayers have never let me down although there is no such thing as instant gratification. We should always remember that our time is not God's time. One of the reasons I wanted to add these prayers to this book is because there are so many folks out there who need them. I have seen folks claim they have demons and all sorts of things crawling around in their bodies. The first thing they should do is seek medical help. The next thing they need to do is cover themselves with the blood of Jesus—nothing evil can stand against that precious blood. Remember: always seek medical help first; root workers are not doctors, so if you're ill, please seek medical attention.

Prayer for the Sick

> *I call on God the Father, God the Son, and God*
> *the Holy Spirit. I pray that _____ be*
> *healed from the top of their head to the bottom of*
> *their feet. That all illnesses be removed, I cover*
> *them with the blood of Jesus that flowed from*
> *our precious Lord's body. Make all that ails them*
> *be driven out by the precious blood of our Lord.*
> *Amen*

To Defeat an Enemy

> *I cover my enemies with the blood of Jesus that*
> *flowed from his right hand, I cover my enemy*
> *with the blood of Jesus that flowed from his left*
> *hand. I cover my enemy with the precious blood*

of Jesus that flowed from his right foot. I cover
my enemy with the precious blood of Jesus that
flowed from his left foot. I cover my enemy with
the precious blood of Jesus that flowed from his
side as the sword pierced his flesh. May all those
who try to harm me and mine be covered with the
blood of Jesus and defeated by the power of his
precious blood. Amen.

Blood of Christ, Inebriate Me!

Blood of Christ, inebriate me!

Inebriate me with Your Love, that I may be
absorbed in Your interests and Your Will.

Absorbed so as to be unmindful of my life and
petty cares.

Unmindful of weariness and pain, heartache and
disappointment.

Heedless of the lash of cruel words and patient
under wrongs. Amen.

O Precious Blood of Jesus

O precious blood of Jesus, infinite price of sin-
ful man's redemption, both drink and layer of
our souls, Thou who dost plead continually the
cause of man before the throne of infinite mercy;
from the depths of my heart, I adore Thee. And
so far as I am able, I would requite Thee for the
insults and outrages which Thee dost continually receive from human beings, and especially
from those who rashly dare to blaspheme Thee.

Who would not bless this blood of infinite value? Who dost not feel within himself the fire of the love of Jesus who shed it all for us? What would be my fate, had I not been redeemed by this divine blood? Who hath drawn from the veins of my Savior, even to the last drop? Ah, this surely was the work of love. O infinite love, which has given us this saving balm! O balm beyond all price, welling up from the fountain of infinite love, grant that every heart and every tongue may be enabled to praise Thee, magnify Thee, and give Thee thanks both now and for evermore. Amen.

Blessed and praised for evermore be Jesus, who hath saved us with His Blood!

Glory to the Blood of Jesus both now and for evermore and through the everlasting ages. Amen.

Prayer to Jesus

We therefore pray Thee, help Thy servants: whom Thou hast redeemed with Thy Precious Blood.

Prayer to the Eternal Father

Eternal Father, I offer Thee the Most Precious Blood of Jesus Christ in atonement for my sins, and in supplication for the holy souls in purgatory and for the needs of holy Church.

Petition

> Lord Jesus Christ, who camest down from heaven
> to earth from the bosom of the Father, and didst
> shed Thy precious blood for the remission of our
> sins: we humbly beseech Thee, that in the day of
> judgment we may deserve to hear, standing at
> Thy right hand: "Come, ye blessed." Who lives
> and reignest for ever and ever. Amen.

Working with the Holy Spirit

The origin of the Holy Trinity can be found in the Bible where Jesus tells his followers to call on the Trinity in Matthew 28 V 19:

> Go ye therefore, and teach all nations, baptizing
> them in the name of the Father, and the Son, and
> of the Holy Spirit.

The Holy Trinity is loaded with power; you could even say that it is "triple action." Old-school workers always begin their work "In the name of God the Father, God the Son, and God the Holy Spirit"; they also end the work with the Trinity because this is a way to nail down the work so it can't be reversed. When you call on God within the Holy Trinity, you are calling on God in all his aspects. In other words you are doing a triple action work.

You can call on the Trinity for protection, success, love, or any situation you may find yourself in. The Trinity is represented by the triangle as well as the number three. So you would say your petition three times a day. I was taught to set the work within the center of a triangle of candles. This is a very powerful way to work with the Trinity. I was also taught to call on the Trinity first, then my ancestors, and then whatever spirit I am gonna petition for help. Nowadays you don't see many conjure workers working with the Trinity. I'm not sure why; maybe they don't know about it or don't realize the power they are missing.

When you need extra power, you can also turn to the Seven Holy Spirits. You may work with them alongside the Holy Trinity or instead of the Trinity, as is best for you.

The Seven Holy Spirits

1. The Spirit of the Lord
2. The Spirit of Wisdom
3. The Spirit of Understanding
4. The Spirit of Counsel
5. The Spirit of Might
6. The Spirit of Knowledge
7. The Spirit of Fear of the Lord

The Sacred Head and Heart of Jesus Prayers

Light a red candle and pray this litany. After each verse pray your petition. Then at the end of the prayer pray your petition. Do this work when everything else has failed.

Litany to the Sacred Head of Jesus

Lord, Have Mercy on Us. Christ, Have Mercy on Us. Lord Have Mercy on Us.

Jesus, Graciously Hear Us.

God the Father of Heaven, Have Mercy on Us.

God the Son, Redeemer of the World, Have Mercy on Us.

God the Holy Ghost. Have Mercy on Us.

Sacred Head of Jesus, Formed by the Holy Ghost in the Womb of the Virgin Mary,

Guide Us in All Our Ways Sacred Head of Jesus, Substantially United to the Word of God,

Guide Us in All Our Ways Sacred Head of Jesus, Temple of Divine Wisdom,

Guide Us in All Our Ways Sacred Heart of Jesus, Center of Eternal Light,

Guide Us in All Our Ways Sacred Head of Jesus, Tabernacle of Divine Knowledge,

Guide Us in All Our Ways Sacred Head of Jesus, Safeguard Against Error,

Guide Us in All Our Ways Sacred Head of Jesus, Sunshine of Heaven and Earth,

Guide Us in All Our Ways Sacred Head of Jesus, Treasure of Science and Pledge of Faith,

Guide Us in All Our Ways Sacred Head of Jesus, Radiant with Beauty and Justice and Love,

Guide Us in All Our Ways Sacred Jesus, Full of Grace and Truth,

Guide Us in All Our Ways Sacred Head of Jesus, Living Witness of Humility,

Guide Us in All Our Ways Sacred Head of Jesus, Reflecting the Infinite Majesty of God,

Guide Us in All Our Ways Sacred Head of Jesus, Center of the Universe,

Guide Us in All Our Ways Sacred Head of Jesus, Object of the Father's Joyous Satisfaction,

Guide Us in All Our Ways Sacred Head of Jesus, Upon Which the Holy Ghost Rested,

Guide Us in All Our Ways Sacred Head of Jesus. Around Which the Glory of Mt. Tabor Shown,

Guide Us in All Our Ways Sacred Head of Jesus, Who Had No Place on Earth on Which to Rest,

Guide Us in All Our Ways Sacred Head of Jesus, Whom the Fragrant Anointing of Magdalen Consoled,

Guide Us in All Our Ways Sacred Head of Jesus, Bathed with the Sweat of Blood in Gethsemane,

Guide Us in All Our Ways Sacred Head of Jesus, Who Wept for Our Sins,

Guide Us in All Our Ways Sacred Head of Jesus, Crowned with Thorns,

Guide Us in All Our Ways Sacred Head of Jesus, Outraged by the Indignities of the Passion,

Guide Us in All Our Ways Sacred Head of Jesus,
Consoled by the Loving Gesture of Veronica,

Guide Us in All Our Ways Sacred Head of Jesus,
Bowed to Earth Which was Redeemed at the
Moment of Death on the Calvary,

Guide Us in All Our Ways Sacred Head of Jesus,
Light of Every Being Born on Earth,

Guide Us in All Our Ways Sacred Head of Jesus,
Our Guide and Our Hope,

Guide Us in All Our Ways Sacred Head of Jesus,
Who Knows All Our Needs,

Guide Us in All Our Ways Sacred Head of Jesus,
Who Gives Us All Graces,

Guide Us in All Our Ways Sacred Head of Jesus,
That Governs All the Motions of the Sacred Heart,

Guide Us in All Our Ways Sacred Head of Jesus,
Whom we Wish to Adore and Make Known
Throughout the World,

Guide Us in All Our Ways Sacred Head of Jesus,
Who Knows All the Secrets of Our Hearts,

Guide Us in All Our Ways Sacred Head of Jesus,
Who Enraptures Angels and the Saints,

Guide Us in All Our Ways Sacred Head of Jesus,
Whom One Day We Hope to Behold Unveiled
Forever,

Guide Us in All Our Ways Sacred Head of Jesus,
We Adore Your Sacred Head; We Surrender
Utterly to All the Decrees of Your Infinite Wisdom.

The Sacred Heart of Jesus

Light a red candle and pray this prayer. Pray one part of the prayer a day for four days. On the fifth day pray the whole prayer.

1. The Word was made Flesh, and dwelt amongst us.

> *Eternal Word, made man for love of us, humbly prostrate at Thy feet, we adore Thee with our whole mind, and with the most profound veneration. To make amends for our ingratitude for so great a benefit, we unite in sincerity of heart with all those who love Thee, and offer Thee, our most humble and affectionate thankgivings. Deeply conscious of that excess of humility, goodness, and sweetness, which we acknowledge in the Divine Heart, we petition Thee for Thy grace to imitate these virtues, so pleasing to Thee.*

> *Say:*

> *Our Father, Who art in heaven,*
> *Hallowed be Thy Name.*
> *Thy Kingdom come.*
> *Thy Will be done,*
> *on earth as it is in Heaven.*
> *Give us this day our daily bread.*
> *And forgive us our trespasses,*
> *as we forgive those who trespass against us.*
> *And lead us not into temptation,*
> *but deliver us from evil. Amen.*
> *Hail Mary, full of grace,*

the Lord is with you.
Blessed are you among women,
and blessed is the fruit of your womb, Jesus.
Holy Mary, Mother of God,
pray for us sinners,
now and at the hour of our death.
Amen.

Glory be to the Father, and to the Son, and to the
Holy Spirit. As it was in the beginning, is now,
and ever shall be, world without end. Amen.

2. He was crucified also for us, suffered under Pontius Pilate, and was buried.

Jesus, our admirable Redeemer, humbly prostrate at Thy feet, we adore Thee with our whole mind, and with the most profound veneration. To testify the grief which we feel for our past insensibility to all the outrages and sufferings which Thy most loving Heart made Thee endure for our salvation, on Thy bitter Passion and death, we unite in sincerity of heart with all those who love Thee, in order that we may thank Thee with our whole soul. We admire the infinite patience and generosity of Thy Divine Heart, and petition Thee to replenish our hearts with that spirit of Christian mortification which will make us embrace sufferings

*courageously and fix our great consolation and
all our glory in Thy cross.*

Say:

*Our Father . . .
Hail Mary . . .
Glory be to the Father . . .*

**3. Thou hast given them bread from heaven, which abounds with
all delights.**

*O Jesus, burning with love for us, humbly pros-
trate at Thy feet, we adore Thee with our whole
mind, and with the most profound veneration. In
order to make atonement for the outrages which
Thy Divine Heart daily receives in the Most
Blessed Sacrament of the Altar, we unite in sincerity of heart with all those who love Thee, and
render Thee the most affectionate thanksgiving.
We love, in Thy Divine Heart, that intensely
burning love which Thou entertainest for Thine
Eternal Father, and humbly beseech Thee to
inflame our hearts with an ardent love of Thee
and of our neighbor.*

Say:

*Our Father . . .
Hail Mary . . .
Glory be to the Father . . .*

*Finally, O most amiable Jesus, we beseech Thee,
by the sweetness of Thy Most Sacred Heart, to*

*convert the sinners, to comfort the afflicted, to
assist the agonizing, and to afford relief to the
holy souls suffering in purgatory. Unite our
hearts in the bonds of true peace and charity,
deliver us from an unforeseen death, and grant
that we may die in holiness and tranquility of
mind.*

Amen.

4. Heart of Jesus, burning with love of us, Inflame our hearts with love of Thee.

*Grant, we beseech Thee, Almighty God, that
we who glory in the most Sacred Heart of Thy
beloved Son, and bear in mind the exceedingly
great benefits of His charity towards us, may
delight in the good conferred on us, and enjoy its
effects, through the same Christ our Lord.*

Amen.

*O Divine Heart of Jesus, I adore Thee with all
the powers of my soul; I consecrate them to Thee
forever, with all my thoughts, words, and actions,
and my whole self. I desire to adore Thee, to love
Thee, and to glorify Thee, in the same manner;
as far as possible, as Thou doest adore love and
glorify Thy Eternal Father. Be Thou, I beseech
Thee, the Restorer of my weakness, and the Pro-
tector of my life, my refuge, and my asylum at
the hour of my death. I conjure Thee, by the sighs
and anguish in which Thou wert immersed for*

me during the whole course of Thy mortal life, to grant me a true contrition for my sins, a contempt of earthly things, an ardent desire of eternal glory, confidence in Thine infinite merits, and final per-severance in Thy grace.

O Heart of Jesus, all love, I offer Thee these hum-ble prayers for myself, and for all those who unite in spirit with me in adoring Thee. Vouchsafe, through Thine infinite goodness, to receive and hear them; above all, for him who among us shall first depart from this mortal life. O amia-ble Heart of my Savior, pour down upon him, in the agony of death, Thine interior consolations; receive him into Thy sacred Wounds; purify him from every defilement in this furnace of love, that Thou mayest grant him admittance into Thy glory, where he may become intercessor, before Thy presence, for all those who remain in this exile.

O Most Holy Heart of my dearly beloved Jesus, I desire to renew and to offer Thee these acts of adoration, and these prayers, every moment I breathe, to the end of my life, for myself, a misera-ble sinner, and for all who are associated with me to adore Thee. I recommend to Thee, O my Jesus, the holy Catholic Church, Thy beloved spouse and our true mother; also, the souls who are undergo-ing Thy justice and all poor sinners, the afflicted, the agonizing, and all mankind. Do not permit Thy Blood, poured out for them, to become useless to them. Vouchsafe, finally, to apply it for the relief of the souls in purgatory, and for those in particular who, during life, were wont devoutly to adore Thee.

O most amiable Heart of Mary, the most pure of all hearts of creatures, and the most replete with the love of the Heart of Jesus, at the same time most merciful towards us, poor sinners, obtain for us, from the Heart of our Redeemer, the graces we ask of thee. Mother of mercy, one look from thee, one movement of Thy Heart, burning with love for that of Jesus, thy divine Son, can fully console us. Grant us, therefore, this favour; and then this divine Heart of Jesus, through the filial love which it bore, and always will bear towards thee, shall not fail to hear and answer our request.

The Sacred Heart of Mary

Light a white candle and pray this prayer for nine days. Pray your petition at the end of the prayer.

Remember. Our Lady of the Sacred Heart, what ineffable power thy divine Son hath given thee over His own adorable Heart. Full of trust in thy merits, we come before thee and beg thy protection. O heavenly Treasurer of the Heart of Jesus, that Heart which is the inexhaustible source of all graces, which mayest open to us at thy good pleasure, in order that from it may flow forth upon mankind the riches of love and mercy, light and salvation, that are contained therein; grant unto us, we beseech thee, the favours which we seek. . . . We can never, never be refused by thee, and since thou art our Mother, O our Lady of the Sacred Heart, graciously hear our prayers and grant our request. Amen.

Prayer to the Virgin Mary

We turn to you for protection, holy Mother of God.

Listen to our prayers and help us in our needs.

Save us from every danger, glorious and blessed Virgin.

Amen

Our Lady of Victory

O Victorious Lady, Thou who has ever such powerful influence with Thy Divine Son, in conquering the hardest of hearts, intercede for those for whom we pray, that their hearts being softened by the ways of Divine Grace, they may return to the unity of the true Faith, through Christ, our Lord. Amen

The Prophets

There were quite a few prophets in the Bible, but we will look at the ones I work with from the Old Testament. First off, you may be wondering what a prophet is. A prophet is a person God chooses to speak his word. God goes directly to the prophet and says what he wants of this person. If you look in Numbers 12 V 1-8, you will see that Aaron and Miriam tried to be the go-between for Moses and God. God put a stop to that fast. God went straight to Moses and told him what he wanted to do.

This also tells us that we don't need a go-between to reach God: he is there waiting. If you look in the book of 1 Kings, you will find out about the Prophet Elijah. God sent Elijah to meet with Ahab. Elijah just showed up one day. You see there was a problem with Jezebel, Ahab's wife. She was ordering God's prophets be put to death. Of course, God didn't appreciate this, so he sent Elijah. It's a whole bunch of drama. Of course, King Ahab wouldn't listen, so God through Elijah brought down a drought—no rain in sight. The drought lasted until God told Elijah it was over.

Are you wondering how Elijah made it through the drought? Well, God had a widow woman and her son help him. In 1 Kings 17 2-7 we see God commanded the widow to help Elijah. We also see that ravens fed him while he waited for God's next move. Elijah also brought the widow's son back from death.

> *2 Then the word of the Lord came to him, saying,*
>
> *3 "Get away from here and turn eastward, and hide by the Brook Cherith, which flows into the Jordan.*

4 And it will be that you shall drink from the brook, and I have commanded the ravens to feed you there."

5 So he went and did according to the word of the Lord, for he went and stayed by the Brook Cherith, which flows into the Jordan.

6 The ravens brought him bread and meat in the morning, and bread and meat in the evening; and he drank from the brook.

7 And it happened after a while that the brook dried up, because there had been no rain in the land.

The Prophet Jeremiah

Jeremiah's life is well-documented; there is more known about his life than any of the other prophets. It is said that Jeremiah was chosen by God before his birth; his book says so in 1 V 5:

Before I formed you in the womb I knew you, before you were born I set you apart; I appointed you as a prophet to the nations.

The prophet Jeremiah can be petitioned for justice, healing, all faith issues, and any other work that you need extra power doing. His name means "God exalts." Anytime you feel crossed up or like a heavy weight is on your shoulders, you can petition Jeremiah to throw the weight off you.

Run Devil Run

Jeremiah 46 V 3-6

3 "Prepare your shields, both large and small, and march out for battle!

4 Harness the horses, mount the steeds! Take your positions with helmets on! Polish your spears, put on your armor!

5 What do I see? They are terrified, they are retreating, their warriors are defeated. They flee in haste without looking back, and there is terror on every side," declares the Lord!

6 "The swift cannot flee nor the strong escape. In the north by the River Euphrates they stumble and fall."

Protection Work

Jeremiah 46 V 27-28

27 "Do not be afraid, Jacob my servant; do not be dismayed, Israel. I will surely save you out of a distant place, your descendants from the land of their exile. Jacob will again have peace and security, and no one will make him afraid.

28 Do not be afraid, Jacob my servant, for I am with you," declares the Lord. "Though I completely destroy all the nations among which I scatter you, I will not completely destroy you. I will discipline you but only in due measure; I will not let you go entirely unpunished."

To Reverse a Jar Work

> *Jeremiah 48 V 12-13*
>
> *12 "But days are coming," declares the Lord,*
> *"when I will send men who pour from pitchers,*
> *and they will pour her out; they will empty her*
> *pitchers and smash her jars.*
>
> *13 Then Moab will be ashamed of Chemosh, as*
> *Israel was ashamed when they trusted in Bethel.*

The Prophet Ezekiel

The prophet Ezekiel was a priest, who was one of the 10,000 Jews taken into exile by Nebuchadnezzar in 597 BCE, when King Jehoiachin was forcibly carried to Babylon. In the fifth year of Jehoiachin's captivity, 593/92, Ezekiel had his first vision by "the river Chebar," a canal near the famous city of Nippur in lower Babylonia (Ezekiel 1 V 1-3). Enigmatic is his statement that this fifth year of captivity was also the "thirtieth year. " It is believed that the prophet refers either to his own age or to that year as the thirtieth year reckoned from the reform which took place during the eighteenth year of Josiah.

Several of the prophet's messages are dated exactly, and the last of these dated prophetic messages was received in the twenty-seventh year of Ezekiel's captivity (29 V 17)—571/70. This leaves Ezekiel with a ministry of at least twenty-two years, from 593/92 to 571/70. However, it is possible that some of his undated prophecies were given at a later time. Hence the year 571/70 must not be considered as necessarily marking the end of his ministry.

To Destroy an Enemy: God's Razor of Judgment

Ezekiel 5 V 1-17

1 "Now, son of man, take a sharp sword and use it as a barber's razor to shave your head and your beard. Then take a set of scales and divide up the hair.

2 When the days of your siege come to an end, burn a third of the hair inside the city. Take a third and strike it with the sword all around the city. And scatter a third to the wind. For I will pursue them with drawn sword.

3 But take a few hairs and tuck them away in the folds of your garment.

4 Again, take a few of these and throw them into the fire and burn them up. A fire will spread from there to all Israel.

5 "This is what the Sovereign Lord says: This is Jerusalem, which I have set in the center of the nations, with countries all around her.

6 Yet in her wickedness she has rebelled against my laws and decrees more than the nations and countries around her. She has rejected my laws and has not followed my decrees.

7 "Therefore this is what the Sovereign Lord says: You have been more unruly than the nations around you and have not followed my decrees or kept my laws. You have not even conformed to the standards of the nations around you.

8 "Therefore this is what the Sovereign Lord says: I myself am against you, Jerusalem, and I will inflict punishment on you in the sight of the nations.

9 Because of all your detestable idols, I will do to you what I have never done before and will never do again.

10 Therefore in your midst parents will eat their children, and children will eat their parents. I will inflict punishment on you and will scatter all your survivors to the winds.

11 Therefore as surely as I live, declares the Sovereign Lord, because you have defiled my sanctuary with all your vile images and detestable practices, I myself will shave you; I will not look on you with pity or spare you.

12 A third of your people will die of the plague or perish by famine inside you; a third will fall by the sword outside your walls; and a third I will scatter to the winds and pursue with drawn sword.

13 "Then my anger will cease and my wrath against them will subside, and I will be avenged. And when I have spent my wrath on them, they will know that I the Lord have spoken in my zeal.

14 "I will make you a ruin and a reproach among the nations around you, in the sight of all who pass by.

15 You will be a reproach and a taunt, a warning and an object of horror to the nations around you when I inflict punishment on you in anger and in wrath and with stinging rebuke. I the Lord have spoken.

16 When I shoot at you with my deadly and destructive arrows of famine, I will shoot to destroy you, I will bring more and more famine upon you and cut off your supply of food.

17 I will send famine and wild beasts against you, and they will leave you childless. Plague and bloodshed will sweep through you, and I will bring the sword against you. I the Lord have spoken."

The Prophet Samuel

In 1 Samuel 2 V 1-10 we see how Hannah prayed to God to be blessed with a child. When she had Samuel, she dedicated him to God. Below you will find Hannah's prayer; this prayer brings forth deliverance from our enemies. If Hannah, who was childless, could pray to God and bring forth a child, then I think her prayer for deliverance would be one that would help deliver folks from their enemies.

You can set up a table with the purple cloth, a cold glass of water, and a reversal candle. Call on the Trinity, then your ancestors, and then call on the prophet Samuel. Light your candle, pray your petition, and then pray Hannah's prayer. Repeat the prayer daily until your candle has burned out.

Hannah's Prayer

1 Then Hannah prayed and said:

"My heart rejoices in the Lord; in the Lord my horn is lifted high.

My mouth boasts over my enemies, for I delight in your deliverance.

2 "There is no one holy like the Lord; there is no one besides you; there is no Rock like our God.

3 "Do not keep talking so proudly or let your mouth speak such arrogance, for the Lord is a God who knows and by him deeds are weighed.

4 "The bows of the warriors are broken, but those who stumbled are armed with strength.

5 Those who were full hire themselves out for food, but those who were hungry are hungry no more.

She who was barren has borne seven children, but she who has many sons pines away.

6 "The Lord brings death and makes alive; he brings down to the grave and raises up.

7 The Lord sends poverty and wealth; he humbles and he exalts.

8 He raises the poor from the dust and lifts the needy from the ash heap; he seats them with princes and has them inherit a throne of honor.

*"For the foundations of the earth are the Lord's;
on them he set the world.*

*9 He will guard the feet of his faithful servants.
But the wicked will be silenced in the place of
darkness "It is not by strength that one prevails;*

*10 those who oppose the Lord will be broken. The
Most High will thunder from heaven; the Lord will
judge the ends of the earth. "He will give strength
to his king and exalt the horn of his anointed."*

The Holy Robe and Holy Stones

The Bible is a powerful book if you know what you are reading. Folks are always looking for power or items to give them power. If you look in Exodus, you might find such information. Not only will you find the instructions for seeking, you will find the instructions for making a Holy Garment. Today these items would be called a robe. It is said that the robe should be made out of blue material. Under the robe white is worn.

If you took the time to read Exodus 28 V 5-14, you would have the knowledge you need to make the holiest of robes to wear during your work. The Bible not only gives instructions on how to make holy oil and other things conjure workers need.

The Ephod

*5 "They shall take the gold, blue, purple, and scar-
let thread, and the fine linen,*

*6 and they shall make the ephod of gold, blue,
purple, and scarlet thread, and fine woven linen,
artistically worked.*

7 It shall have two shoulder straps joined at its two edges, and so It shall be joined together.

8 And the intricately woven band of the ephod, which is on it, shall be of the same workmanship, made of gold, blue, purple, and scarlet thread, and fine woven linen.

9 "Then you shall take two onyx stones and engrave on them the names of the sons of Israel:

10 six of their names on one stone and six names on the other stone, in order of their birth.

11 With the work of an engraver in stone, like the engravings of a signer, you shall engrave the two stones with the names of the sons of Israel. You shall set them in settings of gold.

12 And you shall put the two stones on the shoulders of the ephod as memorial stones for the sons of Israel. So Aaron shall bear their names before the Lord on his two shoulders as a memorial.

13 You shall also make settings of gold,

14 and you shall make two chains of pure gold like braided cords, and fasten the braided chains to the settings.

In Exodus 28 V 15-21 you will find the twelve holy stones. These holy stones are to be placed on a breastplate called the "Breastplate of Justice."

15 "You shall make the breastplate of judgment. Artistically woven according to the workmanship

*of the ephod you shall make it: of gold, blue, pur-
ple, and scarlet thread, and fine woven linen, you
shall make it.*

*16 It shall be doubled into a square: a span shall
be its length, and a span shall be its width.*

*17 And you shall put settings of stones in it, four
rows of stones: The first row shall be a sardius, a
topaz, and an emerald; this shall be the first row;*

*18 the second row shall be turquoise, a sapphire,
and a diamond:*

*19 the third row, a jacinth, an agate, and an
amethyst;*

*20 and the fourth row, a beryl, an onyx, and a
jasper. They shall be set in gold settings.*

*21 And the stones shall have the names of the
sons of Israel, twelve according to their names,
like the engravings of a signet, each one with its
own name; they shall be according to the twelve
tribes.*

Exodus 28 goes on to give more instructions about this holy garment. Then when you move on to Exodus 29 you will be given more
instructions about offerings and such.

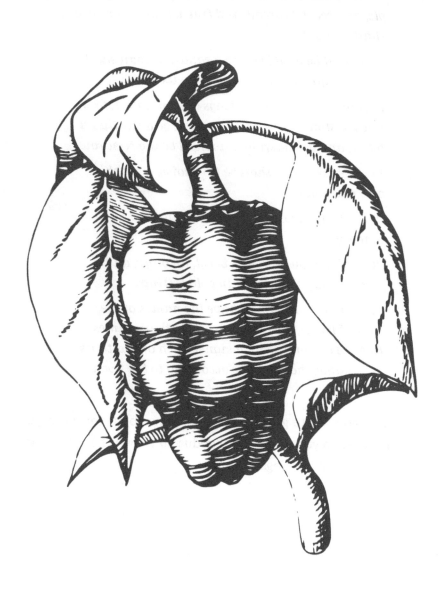

CONCLUSION

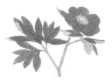

Over the five decades I have been learning, I have had many teachers and elders; I'm still learning. Some of my elders were here for one lesson, as it happens sometimes, and others were with me until they passed on. Each one of them left me with a stepping-stone to grow into the person and worker I am today. For me this started at home with my family. My mama did everything the old way. She gave me a good foundation to grow on even if at the time I didn't know it. I first learned that garlic in sweet oil would cure an earache or that witch hazel would keep the skin clean and clear. I grew up with them; I still use them.

My biggest fear is that this work and knowledge will be lost as elders pass on. No one talks about the power of houseplants anymore. When I was growing up, there were plants in all the homes and on all the door stoops; almost every home had a garden. I wrote this book because the knowledge is being lost or whitewashed—either way it is losing power as folks change the work. Plants are important to this work and to my culture. I hope I have helped keep some part of this knowledge alive with this book.

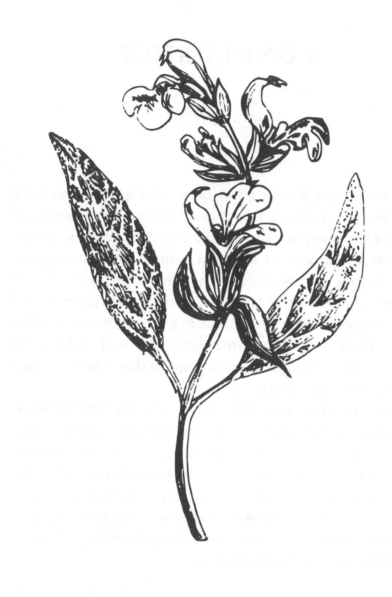

ABOUT THE AUTHOR

Starr Casas holds onto the values of her ancestors. A traditional conjure woman and veteran rootworker of over forty years, Mama Starr is a prolific author and hands-on teacher, who presents workshops throughout the US. She also owns the store Mama Starr's Style LLC in Houston. Find her online at *oldstyleconjure.com* and on Instagram @starrcasas.

TO OUR READERS

Weiser Books, an imprint of Red Wheel/Weiser, publishes books across the entire spectrum of occult, esoteric, speculative, and New Age subjects. Our mission is to publish quality books that will make a difference in people's lives without advocating any one particular path or field of study. We value the integrity, originality, and depth of knowledge of our authors.

Our readers are our most important resource, and we appreciate your input, suggestions, and ideas about what you would like to see published.

Visit our website at *www.redwheelweiser.com*, where you can learn about our upcoming books and free downloads, and also find links to sign up for our newsletter and exclusive offers.

You can also contact us at *info@rwwbooks.com* or at

Red Wheel/Weiser, LLC
65 Parker Street, Suite 7
Newburyport, MA 01950